Amazonian

Gem & Orchid Essences

For Amazonia and its inhabitants

Amazonian

Gem & Orchid
Essences

Andreas Korte
&
Antje and Helmut Hofmann

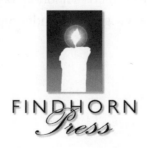

FINDHORN
Press

ISBN 1 899171 91 6

Photographs by Andreas Korte and Peter Kapthammer.
Translated from the German by Carola Splettstößer
and edited by Sandra Kramer.
Cover design and book layout by David Gregson.
Printed by C&C Offset Printing Co., Hong Kong.

Published by
Findhorn Press
The Park, Findhorn
Forres IV36 0TZ
Scotland
tel. +44 (0)1309 690582 • fax. 690036
email thierry@findhorn.org
http://www.gaia.org/findhornpress/

CONTENTS

FOREWORD

THE INDIGENOUS PEOPLES of the Amazon basin often refer to 'The Four Brothers' and express their knowledge through the following maxims:

▶ Never will Amazonia be ruled by humankind. This place is the realm of the Four Brothers: the Forest, the River, the Rain and the Earth.

▶ If one dies, all of them will die, and with them Amazonia.

▶ If you destroy the Forest, the Rain will stop, the Earth will become a desert and the River will dry up.

▶ If there is no Rain, then the Forest will vanish and the Earth will burn and the River will dry up.

▶ If the Earth is pillaged, the Forest will die, the Rain will cease and the River will dry up.

▶ When the River stops flowing, the Forest dies, the Rain stops and the Earth turns to stone.

These Brothers are of divine origin. In its primordial state Amazonia is the sanctuary of the divine on earth, as its natives have always known. This is why, humble of heart, they have always lived with respect for their land and for each of the Brothers.

Today, pride and confusion have led us into an extreme situation. Moreover, human societies are developing on an ever more planetary scale and this means there is less and less of a divide between them, both indirectly and directly, through words, images and trade. And so we are on the threshold of a unified world. As far as the survival of this world is concerned, though, we are on the edge of a precipice.

But Reason and the Muses have not abandoned us entirely, and the protection of the natural environment is humankind's new task. This peaceful crusade will change our mindset and our world-view. It will also help us to modify our production processes, our trading systems and, needless to say, our consumer behaviour, so that we become healthy and happy in harmony with nature.

Humankind is again beginning to perceive the divine essence within nature. The rediscovery of contemplation, the return to revelation and the inner experience of the eternal and the infinite are linked with the liberation of true human nature. Modern society is starting to take an interest in primitive cultures. Furthermore, after introducing a lot of useful and pleasant things to the four corners of the world, it is itself gaining something in exchange. More than one culture is transforming itself after the example of others across time and space.

A marvellous example of this process of change and rediscovery which opens up numerous new perspectives for people is represented by the knowledge that this marvellous book on flower essences presents to the forward-thinking reader.

Flowers are the most beautiful and delicate forms of creation, especially orchids, creatures of light and of the heights of the rainforest, with their fragrance, their subtle energies, their inexhaustible abundance of colours, forms and perfumes. They will begin to enrich the reader's life and also the souls of people around the world.

Moreover, dear reader, these essences make a valuable contribution towards the campaign for the conservation of nature and to protect the culture and life of the indigenous peoples. In effect, to make a financial donation towards the preservation in their original state of the most beautiful places along the equator is an intention and principle intimately linked with the service that humans owe to nature.

Antonio Villa-Lopera
Amacayacu National Park
December 1, 1991

PREFACE

THE IDEA FOR THIS BOOK was born in the sunshine of Tenerife. Andreas Korte, just back from Amazonia, led a workshop on flower essences and then visited Antje and Helmut Hoffman who live on the island. During their conversation they very quickly realised that *the energies of orchids and gemstones could easily be linked*. Amazonia, the source of these gems and flowers, has a very special destiny. In fact, it could be considered the energetic centre of the Earth. The forests of the Amazon are the lungs of the Earth, providing us with oxygen. Therefore the preservation of this region and the help we can give to its flora and fauna are a matter of human survival.

May this book be a gift to you, the reader.

▶ It will introduce you to some of the magnificent gemstones and varieties of crystal from Amazonia and the beauty of the tropical orchids will fill you with delight.

▶ It also gives information on the various orchid and gem essences, how to use them, their characteristics and possible combinations of essences.

May people use these specific energies to raise their vibrations and become aware of their environment, both immediately around them and further afield, thus returning to the source.

We pray that in the beauty and wonders of Amazonia you will find again your own true image.

AMAZONIA

AMAZONIA IS THE LARGEST and most ancient rainforest on our planet. It harbours an infinite number of the most diverse life-forms. Whether you travel by boat along some of the numerous twists and turns of the Amazon river or trek into the deep, dark forest with an Indian guide, you are immediately struck by the density and variety of plants, insects and other animals that live there. This multitude of species has been studied at the University of Bogotà (Colombia). Just as one example, a larger number of species of insect has been found on a single giant tree in the Amazonian forest than in the whole of the UK and Ireland.

Wherever you are in this forest, you feel you are immersed in an intensity of life. The songs of the multicoloured birds mix with the cries of the monkeys and the buzz of the insects — they all harmonise with each other in a magnificent chorus against the backdrop of lush green vegetation. Tree trunks, creepers and aerial roots provide the decor. Wherever you look, you discover new, unknown life-forms: mushrooms in all sizes and superb colours, and butterflies and animals straight out of paradise.

Rainforests have two characteristic features: on the one hand, a three-level structure, each level with its own community of life (biocenosis), and on the other hand, the manner in which the various species of vegetation get their nourishment.

The support and stilt roots of the trees, the bushes and the small palm trees constitute the first dimly-lit level. The second level comprises taller shrubs and trees between five and twenty metres high. On this level live altogether different insects and animals as well as an infinite variety of flowers.

At a height of twenty-five to thirty-five metres, the crowns of the giant trees, bathed in light, form the third level. The treetops are home to an incredibly rich and diverse community of life-forms. Many mammals, birds and amphibians who live there will never touch the ground in their whole lives. And flowers grow in profusion. Seen from above, the forest looks like a huge bouquet. Orchids grow next to other epiphytes on the highest branches, straining towards the sun and the stars.

The second feature unique to the rainforest is that those giant trees are rooted in a layer of humus that is quite shallow, often less than eight centimetres deep. In contrast to other trees, which extract nourishment from the soil and animal droppings by way of their roots, they get their nutrients from on high. The leaves and droppings that fall are quickly decomposed by the billions of bacteria who live in the humus, and the nourishment is absorbed by the roots. In addition, raindrops from the frequent showers carry nutrients all along their descent from leaf to leaf; they reach the soil very slowly so that the trees are continually dripping with water.

The rivulets as well as the numerous rivers and lakes bordered by intensely green vegetation also harbour a great number of life-forms. Depending on the chemical composition of the soil and the speed of the current, the rivers appear clear or muddy. In them live innumerable kinds of fish, amphibians and crustaceans of all sizes and colours. And sometimes the attentive observer will succeed in catching a glimpse of the small pink or large grey dolphins of Amazonia which swim and leap happily in the water.

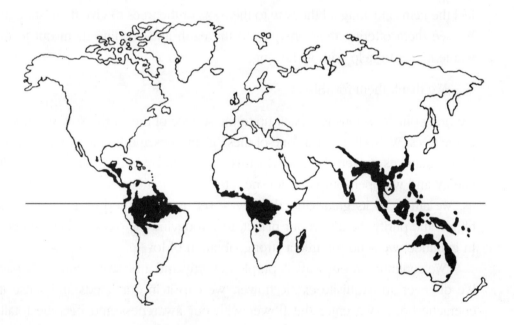

The tropical rainforests — Wolfgang Fremuth
Reproduced by kind permission of BUND

MEDITATION

IF WE TAKE TIME to stop for a while and listen to what is going on inside ourselves, we get in touch with the powerful energies of Amazonia.

We feel our feet in contact with the earth, we sense life pulsating. We attune to the minerals and quartzes which have been formed over thousands of years, and we become one with them. They are everywhere in the earth. They represent the highest energetic expression of the mineral kingdom; they are the fruit of the earth. We allow our consciousness to go down into the ground and make contact with the earth elementals. We visualise the magnificent gemstones and enormous quartzes, and we make contact with their guardians — each gemstone has its own guardian which protects it and ensures that it accomplishes its mission. We feel the gems radiating all the way to the roots of the trees to give them strength. We see them offering their energies to the earth and sending them out to the whole planet to help with its healing.

We thank them for this.

We bring our consciousness back up to the surface of the earth. Now we tune in to the trees. We walk towards one of these giant trees and hug it, or we lean our back against its powerful trunk which is supported by large roots. We sense its energy and we open our consciousness to let this benevolent energy flow into us. We attune to its guardians, the devas. Let us thank the tree for helping to filtrate and purify the air on our planet, for producing the oxygen that we need. In gratitude, we send the tree a strong vibration of love.

We continue on our way. A purple butterfly and a bird of paradise fly past. We discover an exquisite exotic flower. We cup it in our hands and sense its energetic body. We enter the flower with our awareness and become totally immersed in it. We get in touch with the devas of that flower, and we open our heart to let their energy flow in. We start communicating with them, feeling the tremendous warmth and love they radiate. Let's listen to their message. We acknowledge them for giving out their energy into the atmosphere and thus helping living beings to maintain their balance and heal themselves.

We thank them for this.

Our awareness now rises to the crowns of the giant trees and the magnificent orchids growing on their branches. We make contact with the angels of the orchids. We let their wonderful energy sink into us and link us to the invisible world of the angels, and we raise our consciousness to the cosmos. We allow love to flow into us, and we bring it down to our feet and return it to the earth. We become aware of the task of the orchids: to link heaven and earth, humans and angels.

We thank them for this.

Now we bring back our awareness to ground level, and continue on to the banks of the Amazon. We have a good look at the sparkling waters of the longest and most powerful river on earth. We sense the power with which the vast amounts of water make their way down from the Andes all the way to the Atlantic Ocean. We watch the pink dolphins leaping from its waters. We make contact with these intelligent beings who, with their vibrations and their song, speed up the planet's evolution and touch human hearts.

We thank them for this.

Now we make contact with the energy of the river. Its power derives from the essential forces of water, earth, the plants on its banks and the dolphins that swim in its currents. We sense the incredible power with which the river flows — the Amazon is the main artery of our planet's vital energy. Let us be grateful for the gift of life and the balance it brings to the Earth.

We thank it for this.

the INDIANS of AMAZONIA

FOR THE INDIANS OF AMAZONIA, contact with nature and communication with its various energies are as much part of daily life as switching on the television is for us. In the depth of the forest, far away from cities, these men and women lead a way of life still largely protected from the influence of western civilisation.

In Indian culture, trees, animals and stones are looked upon in a fraternal manner, and humans consider themselves part of nature. They have lived in this way for millennia, in harmony with their natural environment and the earth. If, for example, a tree is felled to make a boat, they thank the tree and plant a new one on the same spot in order not to disturb the established natural balance. The Indians are at one with nature, and nature provides them with all that they need.

To cure the sick, they use what they find in their natural surroundings. Their knowledge and experience of stones and plants span generations. For the Indians, physical healing goes hand-in-hand with psychic healing. They work on the fundamental principle that there is no disease but only sick people and bad or negative energy. And if the cause of the disease, which is usually emotional, disappears, the bad energy also vanishes and balance is restored of its own accord. The human organism heals and recovers all its strength and vitality.

Healers called shamans are specially trained to go into a trance and use stones and remedies of plant origin to help people get back into harmony and therefore health. The gemstones they use are most often clear quartz and tropical emerald, a therapeutic stone with a six-pointed-star reflection.

To explore shamanism further would be beyond the scope of this book. However, there is no doubt that western medicine has much to learn from primitive peoples. They demonstrate that we can live in harmony with our environment. Today they urgently need our protection in order to survive. The destruction of their natural habitat is ever-accelerating and the unrelenting advance of our 'civilisation' is, to them, a weapon of mass destruction. We shall address this issue again in the chapter dedicated to the centre of the Earth.

the CARDS

IN THE MIDDLE OF THE BOOK are detachable colour cards that can be used in various ways. The front of each card has a photograph of the gemstone or orchid in question without any distracting caption. On the back is the name of the gemstone or orchid together with the Latin name and a short description.

How to Use the Cards

The cards are particularly useful for choosing an essence. In addition to the intuitive approaches described in the following chapter, the cards can facilitate your inner access to the issue you are focusing on. We suggest you meditate with the cards and attune to the one that most draws you.

Sometimes a flower or a gem will immediately catch your attention. Refer to the description of the flower or gem in this book and absorb the qualities associated with it. Often a certain feeling will come from reading the text, as happens when you watch a beautiful sunset or listen to pleasant music.

You could also spread out all the cards face up, tune in to them and pick out the three or four you like best. Another method is to close your eyes and pass your left — intuitive — hand an inch or so above the cards and attune to the one that attracts you most. Open your eyes and contemplate the picture on the card you have chosen before reading the relevant text and affirmation in the book. Then you can use the corresponding essence in accordance with the methods described.

A note about the affirmations that accompany each gem or orchid essence. These are messages meant for the soul which, if used regularly, will manifest in the subconscious. For the best results, read the affirmation aloud three times in the morning and three times in the evening for a minimum of four weeks. The gem–orchid combinations work gently: the more sensitive the individual, the more marked the transformation. The use and effectiveness of the essences has absolutely nothing to do with quantity, as we are dealing here with bringing body, soul and mind into harmony with subtle cosmic vibrations. Joy, gratitude and trust in the Creator along with regular meditations expedite the healing process.

SELECTING
ESSENCES

WHETHER YOU ARE SELECTING essences for yourself or for someone else, the question arises of which is the best method to follow in making your choice. We have just discussed using the cards but, in that it is impossible to decide on the appropriate essences by purely intellectual means, some other techniques are described below: intuitive selection, radiaesthesia (dowsing), kinesiology and monitoring the pulse.

It may be difficult at first to evaluate the responses from your body. However, the longer you work with each method and thus train your intuition, the more sensitive you will become to your body's reactions.

Intuitive Selection

Whenever you select essences — for yourself or for someone else — there is one fundamental principle that should be observed: free yourself of any egoism which could negatively influence the results of the test.

You have to open up to and trust your own intuition in order to get to the heart of the problem. But who freely acknowledges their weaknesses in our modern culture where 'strength' is everything? It is not easy to see one's own weak points clearly and to work on them, because these are the very aspects of ourselves that we have learned to live with, and this makes it painful to admit to them. Yet recognising one's weak points is the first step towards self-healing. You will be surprised at how quickly you identify them. When you select the essences, you are always led to the key to the problem. In fact, when you are selecting for someone else, you do not necessarily need to know the person or ask them many questions: the intuitive selection process will quickly point out the correct essences and by the same token the relevant issues and their solution. Be prepared to see an astonished expression on the subject's face when you read the description of the essence chosen.

Sensitive people and particularly children have, for the most part, a well developed intuitive sense, which is of great help when it comes to selecting essences. Line up the various essence bottles in front of children and ask them to choose one or two, and they will usually do so quite quickly. On checking, you will be surprised by what they have chosen.

Another intuitive approach is to pass your left hand over the essence bottles and try to feel which bottle attracts you, or what message a particular stone or flower wants to communicate. This method is one that everyone has the ability to use, but many do not dare do so because they lack confidence in their own intuition.

Radiaesthesia (Dowsing)

If you are familiar with using a pendulum, you won't have any problem testing the various essences. It is quite simple: place the pendulum above each bottle, one at a time, then focus on the question, 'Do I need this essence?' Thanks to your previous experience with the pendulum you will already know which direction of rotation means yes and which means no. We recommend that you position the bottles in such a way that you cannot read the labels, in order to eliminate the risk of influencing the process. If you end up selecting several essences, we recommend that you repeat the process with these to narrow down your choice and then read the relevant descriptions in the book.

Kinesiology

This is yet another method based on a muscle test developed by Dr George Goodheart in the USA. It is a very exhaustive test as the subject experiences the reactions in his or her own body. We shall describe the process in detail.

With a friend — and without laughing — try the following:

1. Have your friend remove their watch and stand upright, their left arm hanging loose against their body and their right arm stretched out horizontally (or vice versa if they are left-handed).

2. Stand in front of them; place your right hand on their left shoulder and your left hand on their outstretched arm where their watch would normally be.

3. Tell them that you are going to push down their outstretched arm towards their body. Show them the direction of this movement.

4. Now go back to the original position and ask them to resist your pressure so that their arm remains horizontal.

5. Call out, 'Resist,' and then press their arm down slowly and steadily.

Please note that this is not about strength! It is only about feeling the tension in the muscles, so don't push too hard, just enough to feel the locking of the arm. In the same way, the person being tested must not prevent their arm being pushed down. This is always difficult in the beginning, so practise it several times.

You will learn to recognise the reaction of the body: a 'weak' muscle means that the body does not approve, says no. Conversely, a 'strong' muscle indicates that the body approves, says yes.

Ask your friend to say some agreed-upon sentences and test them immediately after. For example, they can say their name: 'My name is . . .' Test immediately. If the muscle response is strong, their body accepts the affirmation as correct. (With married women, the name of their husband may bring a weak response, which means they do not identify completely with it.) Tell your friend to make up a name and test again: they will react feebly as their body does not approve this affirmation. Try other sentences which you know are true and test these — for instance, name the place where you are. You will see that the body 'knows' what it believes true and what it believes wrong.

Once you have had sufficient practice at this method, you can use it to select essences.

First of all, have your friend ask aloud, 'Do I need any essences?' and test them. If the muscle response is strong, then the answer is yes and you can continue with the exercise. If it is weak, stop the process there. However, bear in mind that the response was true for that moment in time and would not necessarily be true at another time.

If the answer was yes, continue the exercise by testing preselected essences. Place one of the bottles in the hand that is hanging down, ask the person to focus on the question, 'Do I need this essence at this time?' and test the muscle reaction of the other arm. At this stage it is not absolutely necessary for the person to state the question out loud. It is enough for them to keep it in their mind during testing.

You can use the same method to determine the duration of treatment by asking about specific time periods: one week, two weeks, one month and so on.

Monitoring the Pulse

Another method is monitoring the pulse, which originates from Chinese medicine. This form of diagnosis seems difficult at first as it requires great sensitivity of the fingertips, but it is very reliable. Our body reacts to the various stimuli with which it comes into contact as if it had some kind of inner pendulum.

And so you can test the body's reaction to different essences. It is standard practice to take the pulse on the inside of the hand in line with the thumb where there is enough room to place several fingers (but do not use the thumb which has its own pulse). Take hold of the hand of the other person and try to find the pulse.

Normal Pulse   *Rising Pulse*

Next take the essence to be tested in your other hand and slowly bring it closer to the body of the subject. As soon as you come into contact with their astral body (about 40 cm or 16 inches from the physical body), a brief reaction will already become apparent with a change in the pulse, which does not speed up but becomes stronger and more intense. Continue to bring the essence closer until it is some 15 to 20 cm (6 to 8 inches) from the body: once again you will perceive one brief, strong pulsation, as you have just touched the energetic body. The pulse will then remain normal until you touch the physical body, when again you feel a change.

If you are testing a substance that is toxic for the subject and you put it on their skin, the pulse becomes very strong. This violent reaction indicates that the body refuses that substance, and once it is removed the pulse returns to normal.

Test one of the essences (whether a gem, flower or orchid one does not matter): the reaction of the body will be positive. This means it accepts its energy as positive and the pulse quietens down if the essence remains in contact a little longer. As soon as the pulse is back to normal, withdraw the essence from the physical, energetic and astral bodies and notice the strong pulsation: in this way the body indicates its need for that specific energy.

Count the pulsations and repeat the test. If there are more than seven pulsations, this means that the essence is suitable. Test the various essences and you will see that the body knows which are the best ones and which energy it needs at that point in time.

When the selection process identifies several appropriate essences, it remains to consider what is the central theme and to repeat the test in order to narrow the choices down to the one essence to use.

GEMSTONES
and their ESSENCES

The History of Gemstones

Gemstones are an extraordinary gift from the Earth. They developed over millions of years until finally humankind discovered them and brought them into the light of day. They have been treasured by every advanced civilisation, as they have known how to use their secret powers. Ancient traditions mention their therapeutic and harmonising potential for human beings, animals and even plants. Formulae from times past are back in use. For instance, malachite was used to disinfect medical apparatus. Doctors wore emeralds set in rings in order to activate the healing of their patients. Sapphires, rubies, emeralds, amethysts and other very pure and powerful gems enhanced the appearance of both spiritual and temporal dignitaries and also fed their inspiration.

Eight hundred years ago, Hildegarde of Bingen compiled clear information on the medicinal use of plants and minerals. Her teachings show that body, soul and mind are one entity and should be treated as such. But a large portion of past tradition and knowledge has been lost. Having abandoned holistic thinking, scientists of recent centuries have instead focused on analysing and examining matter. But today, at the dawn of the age of Aquarius, holistic thinking is making a reappearance. Gemstones are gaining ever more importance in the therapeutic process. Extracts of plants, flowers and gems are a relatively easy-to-use method for aiding the healing process.

The Action of Gemstones

Contrary to popular belief, gemstones are not inert matter. They grow and develop organically, albeit much more slowly than plants, animals and humans. Geologists have identified seven different models of growth for gemstones, called crystalline systems: isometric, tetragonal, hexagonal, trigonal, orthorhombic, monoclinic, triclinic.

These seven systems allow us to classify all gemstones apart from amorphous stones, which do not have a regular, crystalline structure, such as amber, opal, obsidian, moldavite and jet.

When crystals are charged with energy, they react in an interesting manner: they translate that energy into another form. For instance, an electric current will be transformed into vibrations and similar intensities will result in identical vibrations. This is the mechanism used in modern quartz watches and clocks. If a crystal is compressed, the energy is transformed into electricity. This reaction is now used in cigarette lighters to produce the initial spark.

So crystals transform the energy they receive. If we wear or carry a gem, our own energy enters the stone and is therefore transformed. This is easy to try out with a clear quartz, whatever its shape: place it in your hand, relax and observe your reactions. Do you feel a pulsating energy? Do you have a sense of calm and balance? Most people can immediately perceive the change in themselves.

This transformation of energy is only one of the actions carried out by gemstones. Just as human beings have more than one gift or characteristic, so do stones have other properties too. They act through their colours, their chemical composition, their shape and crystalline system, their electromagnetic vibration, their transparency and their hardness.

Colour

Colour is the language of light. Colours come from light. White light is made up of electromagnetic vibrations comprising all colours. If a part of white light is absorbed, its spectrum decreases and we see colours as a result. Light can either pass through a gem or be partially absorbed. A colourless stone lets all the light pass through it, whereas a black stone absorbs it all. Amethyst, for instance, absorbs all colours except purple. Purple is a very short wavelength vibration and acts mostly in the spiritual realms, whereas the wavelength of red is twice as long and acts mostly on the physical level. Body, soul and mind can be harmonised by means of their missing colours, a process that is used in chromatherapy. Gems also act through their luminous colours, which speak to people's feelings in particular. In the chapter 'Chakras and Gemstones' we shall see how the colours correspond to the energetic centres of the human body.

Chemical Composition

A large number of gems consist mainly of silica, but there are many other components as well. Human beings can receive the substances they lack in a subtle form, diluted in the essence which is applied to the skin. For instance, haematite contains iron, pearls are rich in calcium, malachite contains copper and clear quartz is made up of silica. The chemical mix acts mainly on the bloodstream but affects the whole of the human body.

Shape and crystalline system

The shape of minerals is often symbolic and this has a variety of implications for human beings. A stone's shape is often altered or accentuated by being cut in order to bring out the colour, scintillation or fire of the gemstone. The shape and crystalline system influence our cellular consciousness and our spiritual outlook.

Electromagnetic vibrations

Thanks to Kirlian photography these can be observed and are different for every stone. They could be regarded as the aura of the stones and they affect the human energetic body.

Transparency

The degree of transparency of stones varies. Clear stones affect the thought processes, translucent stones affect all energy-generating organs such as the heart and the lungs, while opaque stones affect all organs of transformation such as the stomach and intestines.

Hardness

Hard stones like diamond, ruby, sapphire and topaz reinforce and strengthen the personality and the thought processes. Soft stones such as calcite, fluorite, turquoise and azurite soften aspects of the personality which are too rigid and help increase tolerance.

Health is a perfect state of balance. Gemstones, with their beautiful colours, shapes and sparkle, allow us to achieve this balance and attain harmony in a particularly agreeable manner.

using GEMSTONES

WE CAN CHOOSE from a wide variety of ways to make use of the beneficial properties of gemstones. Here are some of them:

Form in which used

- ▶ Uncut
- ▶ En cabochon
- ▶ Fashioned (for example, rose cut, cross cut or table cut)
- ▶ Tabular
- ▶ Gem water
- ▶ Gem essence
- ▶ Gem cream

Methods of use

- ▶ Lay out the stones in the form of a mandala (to use as either a symbolic image or an aid to meditation)

- ▶ Wear the stones as jewels if set in appropriate metals such as gold, silver, copper or platinum

- ▶ Meditate with gemstones

- ▶ Use the gem essences either internally or externally

- ▶ Apply some gem cream

Cleansing Gemstones

Before using gemstones in therapy, in making essences or on oneself, it is essential to cleanse them. There are many methods for doing this, including the following, which we have found the most effective and easiest to use:

1. Place the stone under running water for a few minutes, or alternatively leave it for at least two hours in a container with about a litre (two pints) of water.

2. Leave the stone in sea salt for two to three days and then rinse it in clear water.

3. Leave the stone for a minimum of two hours in a distilled water solution to which has been added either three tablespoons of sea salt or five tablespoons of cider vinegar.

4. Leave the stone for two days in soil that is free of fertilisers and then rinse in clear water.

5. Hold the stone in your cupped hands and visualise a mountain stream or a waterfall washing away from the stone all the impurities and the programming that accompanies them.

Do not use methods two or three with delicate or sensitive stones such as pearls, corals, malachite, azurite, turquoise, chrysocolla or selenite.

CHAKRAS and GEMSTONES

HERE WE DESCRIBE the main energy centres of the body plus two secondary centres and classify the stones according to colour, crystalline structure and ability to stimulate each chakra. The chakras are the points in the body that regulate the intake and output of energy.

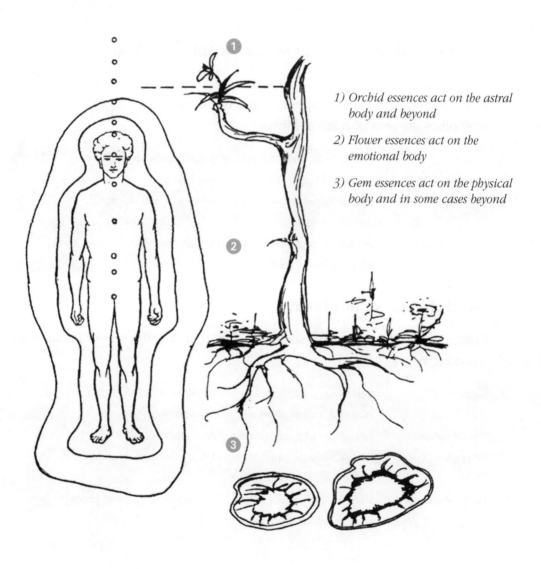

1) *Orchid essences act on the astral body and beyond*

2) *Flower essences act on the emotional body*

3) *Gem essences act on the physical body and in some cases beyond*

▶ First chakra: root (or base) chakra

Situated between the coccyx and the sacrum, it receives energy from the earth. It symbolises harmony with the earth, fighting spirit, courage and the instinct for survival.

Colour	red (e.g. ruby, garnet, red coral, agate, haematite, flint)
Crystal system	isometric (e.g. pyrite, garnet, fluorite)
Properties	harmony with the earth, security, sense of responsibility, sexuality, life force and courage
Energy imbalances	insufficient powers of recovery, aggressiveness, disorganised life, excessive dependence on material objects, selfishness, poor metabolism, fear of living

▶ Second chakra: sacral (or sexual or spleen) chakra

Situated between the fifth lumbar vertebra and the sacrum, it receives energy from the sun. It regulates digestion and elimination. The second chakra also symbolises the area of relationships.

Colour	orange (e.g. carnelian, fire opal, padparadscha)
Crystal system	tetragonal (e.g. rutile, zircon, apophyllite)
Properties	joie de vivre, group consciousness, exhilaration, growth and creativity
Energy imbalances	existential angst, fear of contact, guilt feelings, infectious disease and emotional coldness

▶ Third chakra: solar plexus

Situated under the sternum, it stimulates digestion. It is the seat of intuition and individuality.

Colour	yellow (e.g. sherry-yellow topaz, citrine, tiger's eye, amber, heliodor, yellow diamond, rutilated quartz)
Crystal system	hexagonal (e.g. aquamarine, beryl, emerald)
Properties	seat of feelings, of creativity, of will-power, of discrimination, of focusing and of thinking
Energy imbalances	thirst for power, depression, dissatisfaction, mistrust, jealousy, pain (stomach, liver, gall-bladder)

► Fourth chakra: heart chakra

Situated at the level of the sternum, it ensures the regulation of the heart, the thymus and the circulation. It is the seat of love and tolerance.

Colour	green (e.g. moss agate, aventurine quartz, emerald, chrysoprase, peridot, malachite, jade, dioptase)
Colour	pink (e.g. rose quartz, rhodochrosite, rhodonite, kunzite, pink coral, rose tourmaline)
Crystal system	trigonal (e.g. agate, clear quartz, citrine, dioptase, haematite, moss agate, tourmaline)
Properties	unity, love, reconciliation, tolerance, purity, joy in contact and harmony
Energy imbalances	intolerance, fanaticism, disturbed receptivity, insensitivity, indifference, heart and circulation problems, immune system deficiencies, lung diseases and thymus problems

► Fifth chakra: throat chakra

Situated in the larynx in the middle of the neck, it regulates the lymph, the thyroid gland, verbal expression of feelings and vibrations.

Colour	pale blue (e.g. turquoise, aquamarine, chalcedony, moonstone, chrysocolla)
Crystal system	orthorhombic (e.g. alexandrite, chrysoberyl, celestite, peridot, topaz)
Properties	expression of feelings in words, music, painting and writing. Truth, knowledge, inspiration and creativity.
Energy imbalances	difficulties with language and expression, gossip, thyroid problems, imperious behaviour and distortion of intuition

► Sixth chakra: frontal chakra or third eye

Situated between the eyebrows, it regulates the thought processes and intuition.

Colour	indigo (e.g. lapis lazuli, sodalite, azurite, sapphire)
Crystal system	monoclinic (e.g. azurite, charoite, kunzite, malachite)
Properties	seat of spiritual vision and intuition, ability to concentrate, wisdom, extrasensory perception, clear image of goal
Energy imbalances	insecurity, lack of control, chaos, weariness with life, presumptuousness, exhaustion, visual problems and memory loss

▶ **Seventh chakra: crown chakra**

This is linked to the epiphysis and is situated on the crown of the head. It expresses spirituality and cosmic unity.

Colour	purple (e.g. amethyst, sugilite, fluorite, purpurite, charoite
Crystal system	triclinic (e.g. amazonite, labradorite, rhodonite)
Properties	contact with the Higher Self, spirituality, awareness, access to the subconscious
Energy imbalances	lack of enthusiasm, depression, fear of death, hyperactivity, migraines and headaches

▶ **The secondary chakras of the hands and feet**

In the palms of the hands are the chakras that regulate energy exchanges with the outside.

Colour	white (e.g. clear quartz, diamond, zircon)
Crystal system	triclinic (e.g. cyanite, labradorite)
Properties	harmony, exchange of information and energy, clarity, expression of energy
Energy imbalances	insufficient expression, blocked circulation in the hands, lack of sensitivity

On the soles of the feet are the chakras that link the body and all the chakras with the earth.

Colour	black (e.g. onyx, obsidian, black tourmaline, smoky quartz)
Crystal system	isometric (e.g. garnet, diamond, pyrite, spinel)
Properties	connection with the earth, stability, resilience, steadfastness
Energy imbalances	hiding from the world, neglect of the physical, disharmony, leg problems

the HIGHER CHAKRAS

ONGOING EVIDENCE about the energy centres in the skull and above shows that these higher chakras link us to our as-yet unconscious creative faculties, to our Higher Self and to divine awareness. Now, at the dawn of the Age of Aquarius, we are becoming aware of those gifts and potentials that will allow us to meet the specific demands of our times and tap new forms of energy. Here are some stones that can help to support and stimulate those chakras:

▶ The colours of cyanite range from blue to green, sometimes with yellow, pink or white streaks fanning out in the crystals. Cyanite brings light and enlightenment to body and spirit, shatters ancient and outdated ways of thinking and facilitates the emergence of higher thought-forms.

▶ Moldavite, an amorphous, green, clear stone, is the result of the fusion of a meteorite with the rocky ground of the Earth. It is of help to human beings who feel they do not belong on Earth and allows them to adjust. Additionally, it opens us up to new ways of thinking and prepares us to make contact with extraterrestrial life-forms.

▶ Selenite (crystal gypsum) is a translucent crystal that grows in the form of small rods. It brings light to our feelings and stabilises them. Selenite helps to integrate the highest aspects of light into matter.

▶ Blue Tourmaline also grows in the form of small rods. It brings light to consciousness and facilitates the assimilation of new knowledge.

▶ Blue star sapphire shows a star on its surface. It fosters evolution of the mind and improves the power of concentration. Just like the rays of the star focus at its centre, thoughts are directed towards the essential issue of the moment.

▶ Calcite comes in many colours (white, yellow, orange, pink, green, gold, blue, grey and red) and ranges from translucent to opaque. It brings spiritual understanding to daily life, and is also of great help in difficult times.

MAKING & BOTTLING
the essences

THE ESSENCES ARE CONCENTRATES of flowers or gemstones and in this form their energy is more accessible as the active elements easily penetrate the physical and subtle bodies and can start acting immediately.

The preparation of gem essences requires:

▶ a gemstone for the selected essence

▶ a crystal cup (either a geode or a plain undecorated glass)

▶ distilled water

▶ some gauze to cover the cup

▶ surgical spirit to wipe the container

▶ sunshine: if possible choose a time of a waxing or full moon

▶ possibly four to eight clear quartz needles

The gemstones used for the preparation of the essences must not contain any foreign mineral substance and should not, as far as possible, have been cut. In this case 'foreign' means not belonging to the same group — for example, calcite that has grown on an amethyst. Whenever possible, try to use high-quality specimens with intense colours.

First of all, the stones are cleansed, as described on pages 23-4, and then left in the sun for one to two hours.

In order to obtain a high-quality essence, you yourself need to be healthy and feel joyful and harmonious. Filled with love, make spiritual contact with the stone that you are planning to use, and then proceed as follows:

1 Take the container you have chosen and sterilise it, either with boiling water or surgical spirit.

2 Place the stone in the cup and add about half a litre (³/4 pint) of distilled water.

③ Cover the container with gauze and place it in the open air in the sun.

④ In order to activate the process, place four to eight clear quartz needles near the container at equal distances from each other and pointing towards the glass or geode.

⑤ Visualise yourself surrounded by light. Similarly, imagine the container surrounded by light. When breathing in, consciously draw in light and cosmic energy. When breathing out, let go of everything that is heavy, murky, dark. Repeat this until a light with a golden border surrounds the whole of your physical body and the container with the stone — either in its own light bubble or as part of yours. Then ask the guardians of the stone for their help in charging the water with its energy. Focus intensely on the transmission of energy and information from the stone to the water.

⑥ Leave the container in the open air in the sun for a minimum of eight hours, preferably for a full twenty-four hours; if possible, this should be during a waxing or full moon. Or prepare a container with the stone and distilled water, hermetically seal it and place it in the open air for a minimum of a week during a waxing to full moon.

⑦ In order to preserve the essence for long-term use, place in small sterilised bottles (20-30 ml or up to 1 fl. oz.) and fill them with half essence and half good-quality brandy. Seal and label (for example, Diamond Mother Tincture). Keep the bottles in a cool, dark place five centimetres (two inches) apart, away from any electrical wires, sockets or apparatus.

E using the SSENCES

TAKING ESSENCES allows us to benefit from the specific properties of gemstones, such as their colour and trace elements (for example, silica, magnesium, calcium, lithium and various metals). Humans, animals and plants can be helped by this subtle contribution to well-being.

Internal use

The mother tincture must be diluted before use. Half-fill a small dropper bottle (20-30 ml or up to 1 fl. oz.) with spring or mineral water and top up with brandy. Then add a few drops of the mother tincture. Shake well.

Before taking a dose, shake the bottle again ten times to energise the essence. For short-term use (i.e. less than three days) one can dilute the mother tincture drops in water. However, for longer-term use, brandy is indispensable.

External use

Many gem essences work well when used externally. Clear Quartz essence can be added to all mixtures. This essence is particularly potent in skin ointments and creams. Emerald, Aquamarine and Amazonite essences can be used in a similar fashion.

Emerald, Aquamarine or Clear Quartz essences can be added to the water of compresses aimed at relieving eye inflammation. Clear Quartz essence has a refreshing action on the head and the whole body.

It is also possible to use the essences directly on the skin, on the reflex zones, the chakras or the acupuncture meridians. A cream mixed with the appropriate gem or orchid essences is particularly good for massaging the face and the reflex zones of the hands and feet. (See the section on gem and orchid creams.)

For plants and animals

To allow our domestic animals and houseplants to receive light and love and to benefit from the energies of the essences, we recommend a mixture of the

Amazonas and Clear Quartz essences. Two drops in the drinking water or the watering can at regular intervals for four to seven days is sufficient.

Combinations

Gem and orchid essences combine easily according to need. Dosage directions must be precisely defined and intake rhythm followed scrupulously. Pairings of orchids and gemstones, together with their respective affirmations, are clearly indicated in this book. However, if your own tests reveal a different match, trust your choice.

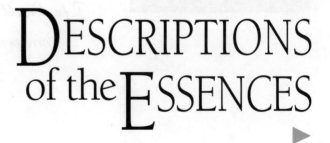

DESCRIPTIONS
of the ESSENCES
▶

AMAZONITE

Crystal system:	Triclinic
Hardness:	6.0–6.5
Chemical formula:	$K(AlSi_3O_8)$
Composition:	Potassium aluminium silicate
Transparency:	Opaque to translucent
Colour:	Green, blue-green
Sign of the zodiac:	Virgo
Element:	Air
Chakras:	Heart, third eye, crown

▶ Amazonite is an opaque, green to bluish-green feldspar. Its name derives from the Amazon river.

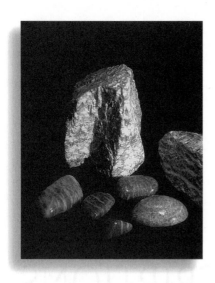

Amazonite essence

This essence balances the nervous system and muscle tone. Taken three times daily it improves the body's assimilation of potassium and calcium.

It fosters increased awareness of the various layers of our personality and harmony with our surroundings. It makes access to the real nature of gems and plants easier.

Affirmation:
I feel well within the flow of life.

Corresponding orchid: Deva Orchid

AMETHYST

Crystal system:	Trigonal
Hardness:	7.0
Chemical formula:	SiO_2
Composition:	Silica
Transparency:	Transparent
Colour:	Purple, pale red-purple
Sign of the zodiac:	Pisces, Virgo, Aquarius, Capricorn
Element:	Air
Chakras:	Third eye, crown

▶ Amethyst is a gemstone of either a pale- or dark-purple colour with well formed tips. Sometimes it grows in light-purple groups or in the shape of a sceptre.

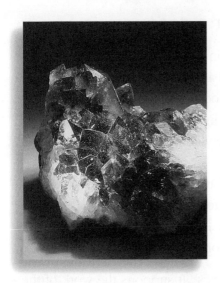

Amethyst essence

With its soft and soothing vibration this essence facilitates getting in touch with the unconscious mind and soul level. It helps balance a body suffering from disrupted sleep and an exaggerated focus on mental activity, which can manifest in headaches, migraine, neuralgia, arthritis and stress.

Amethyst strengthens the endocrine glands and the nervous system, and also opens up access to the intuitive and dream level.

Taking some Amethyst essence is an ideal preparation for meditation; it is, however, sufficient just to hold the essence bottle in your hand whilst meditating. You will sleep better and the effects of stress will be eliminated.

Spiritual development will be enhanced, as the essence particularly stimulates and opens the sixth and seventh chakras.

Affirmation:
I am filled with light and love.

Corresponding orchid: Psyche Orchid

AQUAMARINE

Crystal system:	Hexagonal
Hardness:	7.5–8.0
Chemical formula:	$Al_2Be_3(Si_6O_{18})$
Composition:	Beryllium aluminium silicate
Transparency:	Transparent to opaque
Colour:	Light blue, blue-green
Sign of the zodiac:	Gemini, Pisces, Aries
Element:	Water
Chakras:	Throat, third eye

▶ Aquamarine is a soft, transparent light blue to blue-green. It grows as hexagonal column-shaped prisms.

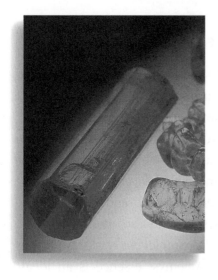

Aquamarine essence

Its name — in Latin: water of the sea — gives a clue to its action: in a gentle but persistent manner it washes away blockages and obstacles; it purifies, clears and brings light into the body and aura. It is particularly active within the area of the neck and head.

It greatly enhances the capacity for verbal self-expression. Your feelings flow to the surface more easily. Any stress and burden can be shared with others and therefore reduced.

Aquamarine essence soothes and 'calms the waves'. It supports the work of the body's purifying organs such as liver, kidneys, spleen and lymph. The activity of the brain calms down, and thoughts become lucid. Aquamarine refreshes the eyes and aids 'intuitive vision'.

Affirmation:
I can express my feelings in a free and loving way.

Corresponding essence: Amazonas

CITRINE

Crystal system:	Trigonal
Hardness:	7.0
Chemical formula:	SiO_2
Composition:	Silica
Transparency:	Transparent
Colour:	Yellow, reddish brown
Sign of the zodiac:	Gemini, Aries, Leo, Libra
Element:	Air
Chakras:	Sacral, solar plexus, third eye, crown

▶ Most citrines are actually heat-treated amethysts or smoky quartzes. At 450°C the colour of an amethyst changes to light yellow and at 550–560° it changes from dark yellow to reddish brown. Smoky quartz becomes the colour of citrine at 300–400°C. Natural citrines are rather pale yellow and much more rare.

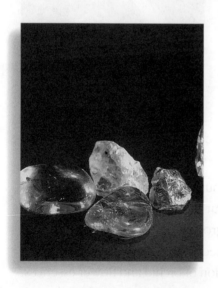

Citrine essence

This essence balances the emotional level in the solar plexus and reinforces self-confidence, intuition and sense of community. It allows us to recognise the beauty and joy in life and gives us courage to start anew.

On the physical level it stimulates digestion, blood circulation, the purifying organs of the body and the nerves. It activates the third eye and crown chakras, which helps to balance intuition and mind. It strengthens the connection with the Higher Self.

Affirmation:
Joy surges through me and opens all doors.

Corresponding orchid: Chocolate Orchid

CLEAR QUARTZ

Crystal system:	Trigonal
Hardness:	7.0
Chemical formula:	SiO_2
Composition:	Silica
Transparency:	Transparent
Colour:	None
Sign of the zodiac:	All
Element:	Water
Chakras:	All

▶ Clear quartz grows in hexagonal prisms. It has piezo-electric and pyro-electric qualities, which means that when the crystal is submitted to heat or pressure it renders the energy of these in an altered form. The energy of pressure becomes electricity — a principle used, for example, in modern cigarette lighters. This allows a transformation, increase and concentration of energy. The same applies to the energies of the physical body, which are also cleared and activated by clear quartz. The crown chakra can be stimulated 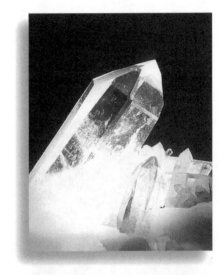 and opened with its help, thereby improving your connection with your Higher Self, provided that you are willing to accept your inner guidance.

Clear quartzes often grow in caves in groups or as outgrowths of the underlying rock. Small sphere-shaped 'cavities' lined with crystals are called geodes. Geodes of clear quartz are perfect for the production of orchid and flower essences. The clear quartz conducts the plant's vibration into the water and anchors it there. This method is very subtle and does not damage the plant. It makes sure that no vibration of pain, which occurs when picking plants, will be conducted into the essence.

Certain crystals have a point at each end: these contain all the properties of clear quartz in a stronger form and they balance polarities. They harmonise, connect the chakras and dissolve tension.

Clear Quartz essence

This essence has a purifying and detoxifying effect on body and soul. It tidies up and clarifies energies that have been absorbed. Its radiant vibration enhances and protects the body's own energy field (the aura). It facilitates intuition and access to the Higher Self. Within the physical body Clear Quartz essence helps the functioning of skin, hair and bones with its cleansing and detoxifying properties. It also stimulates and harmonises the endocrine glands, lungs, heart and nervous system.

Affirmation:
My Higher Self is my guide.

Corresponding orchid: Higher Self Orchid

DIAMOND

Crystal system:	Isometric
Hardness:	10
Chemical formula:	C
Composition:	Crystallised carbon
Transparency:	Transparent
Colour:	None, yellow, brown, blue, pink, black
Sign of the zodiac:	Aries, Taurus, Leo
Element:	Fire
Chakras:	Third eye, crown

▶ The diamond derives its name from its hardness (Greek: *adamas* — invincible). The carbon of which it is composed is the hardest matter known. It may be colourless or can appear in a variety of colours such as yellow, brown, blue, pink and black. Due to its sparkle and refraction it is seen as the epitome of all gemstones. It grows in various shapes such as octahedra and cubes.

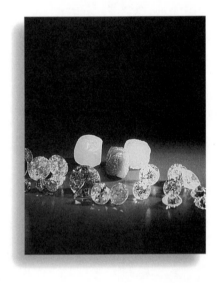

Diamond essence

Diamond essence casts light onto the shadows of the soul. Clarity and insight enhance self-realisation. It purifies the mind as well as the body. When one is meditating and channelling, Diamond essence is an aid to lucid transmission and a good connection with the Higher Self and the cosmos. It renders truth visible and tears down the boundaries and limitations we have erected between ourselves and others. We are able to look into our innermost being.

Affirmation:
I love myself and others, even though I recognise our weaknesses.

Corresponding orchid: Channelling Orchid

ELESTIAL QUARTZ

Crystal system:	Trigonal
Hardness:	7.0
Chemical formula:	SiO_2
Composition:	Silica
Transparency:	Transparent to opaque
Colour:	Colourless, light to dark brown
Sign of the zodiac:	All
Element:	Fire
Chakras:	Feet, base, solar plexus, crown

▶ Elestial quartz is usually light to dark brown, similar to smoky quartz. It often ends in one point only; sometimes it has several points which are flattened and look like they have been compressed.

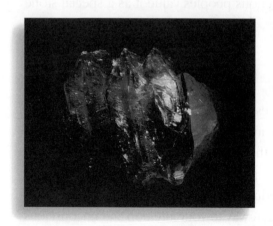

Elestial Quartz essence

This essence demands a lot of you. It should be taken carefully and in a very conscious way. It is very clear in letting you know whenever 'your' truth is out of step with universal truth. You should be prepared for that, for it gives rise to processes of transformation aimed at re-establishing harmony.

As you let go of old patterns and beliefs there may be some painful and difficult steps in store for you. Blockages in your energetic centres will be dissolved, the gall bladder will rid itself of old, bottled-up anger and cerebral activity will come into balance. Elestial Quartz essence facilitates the changes necessary for the next level of development.

Affirmation:
I set free my pent-up energies and emotions, and I open myself up to new experiences.

Corresponding orchid: Aggression Orchid

EMERALD

Crystal system:	Hexagonal
Hardness:	7.5–8.0
Chemical formula:	$Al_2Be_3(Si_6O_{18})$
Composition:	Beryllium aluminium silicate
Transparency:	Transparent to opaque
Colour:	Green
Sign of the zodiac:	Taurus, Gemini, Aries
Element:	Air
Chakras:	Heart, third eye

▶ Emerald grows in stem-shaped hexagonal prisms and gets its colour from chromium or vanadium. Its typical magnificent green varies from transparent to opaque. The tropical emerald with its inner six-pointed star is a renowned variety that comes from Colombia, where the indigenous peoples value it as a special stone for healing.

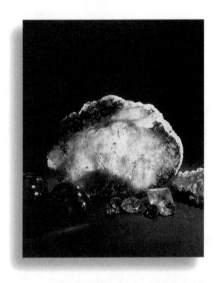

Emerald essence

Emerald essence opens your heart to life's great diversity and helps you to accept more easily energies that do not correspond with your own thought patterns. Love as a feeling of connectedness with all fills your heart. The third eye, the gateway to your intuition and unconscious capacities, is activated. Your expanded understanding stimulates cell growth. Old patterns dissolve and your connection with your Higher Self becomes clearer.

The loving, harmonious vibration of this essence refreshes and regenerates body and mind. It strengthens the personality and quells or eliminates anxieties.

Affirmation:
Love dissolves all fear.

Corresponding Orchid: Venus Orchid

HAEMATITE

Crystal system:	Trigonal
Hardness:	5.5–6.5
Chemical formula:	Fe_2O_3
Composition:	Ferrous oxide
Transparency:	Opaque
Colour:	Black, with a silver sheen
Sign of the zodiac:	Aries, Aquarius
Element:	Fire
Chakra:	Base

▶ Haematite grows mostly in kidney-shaped lumps or in slabs of crystal. The native North Americans utilise these haematite lumps as magic stones. Although it appears black with a silvery sheen, it is actually red. When the stone is cut, the cooling water is dyed blood red — whence its name (Greek: *haima* = blood); in some languages it is also known as 'bloodstone'.

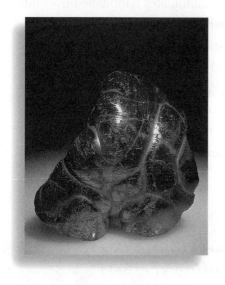

Haematite essence

This essence energises the blood and increases oxygenation. It refreshes and enlivens the body, skin and organs and stimulates the mind and intuition. On a psychological level it strengthens self-confidence and encourages greater lucidity of thought and expanded mental capacity. Your range of awareness increases, and you begin to understand that the only limits are those you have created yourself. The abundance of the universe is on offer. Body, mind and soul achieve a better balance. Your own feelings become clearer and more comprehensible.

Affirmation:
The abundance of life stimulates me.

Corresponding orchid: Horn of Plenty Orchid

MOONSTONE

Crystal system:	Monoclinic
Hardness:	6.0–6.5
Chemical formula:	$K(AlSi_3O_8)$
Composition:	Potassium aluminium silicate
Transparency:	Transparent
Colour:	Colourless, yellow, pale blue, orange
Sign of the zodiac:	Cancer, Libra, Scorpio
Element:	Water
Chakras:	Solar plexus, throat, third eye

▶ Moonstone is a colourless, yellow, pale blue, pink or orange feldspar. It has a bluish, pearly sheen.

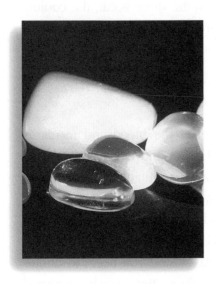

Moonstone essence

Moonstone essence stimulates lymphatic flow and therefore the detoxification of the body. It enhances one's dreamy, inspirational and feminine aspects. Self-expression and creativity are strengthened. You recognise and accept your feelings to a greater extent, and become more aware of dreams expressing your emotional life. In addition, you understand the feelings of others more easily.

Affirmation:
I give attention to my feelings and accept them, and I have a deeper understanding of others.

Corresponding orchid: Inspiration Orchid

OLIVINE

Crystal system:	Orthorhombic (prisms)
Hardness:	6.5–7.0
Chemical formula:	$(Mg, Fe)_2SiO_4$
Composition:	Magnesium iron silicate
Transparency:	Transparent
Colour:	Olive green, yellowish green
Sign of the zodiac:	Virgo, Leo, Scorpio, Sagittarius
Element:	Fire
Chakras:	Solar plexus, heart

▶ Olivine is usually yellow–green, olive green (whence its name) or brownish and it grows in short rhombic prisms. It is also called peridot or chrysolite.

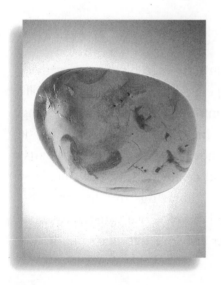

Olivine essence

Olivine essence emits a light, joyous vibration. Joy, which we also recognise in others, radiates in and out of us like the sun and allows us to express our feelings more easily.

The heart and solar plexus chakras and their corresponding organs are stimulated and cleansed and open up to joy and love. Any tension and strain is dissolved, which aids the circulation of the body's energies.

Affirmation:
My joy radiates outwards to everything around me.

Corresponding orchid: Fun Orchid

ROSE QUARTZ

Crystal system:	Trigonal
Hardness:	7.0
Chemical formula:	SiO_2
Composition:	Silica
Transparency:	Transparent
Colour:	Pink
Sign of the zodiac:	Taurus, Libra
Element:	Water
Chakras:	Heart, crown

▶ Rose quartz grows in various micro-crystalline forms, more rarely as a crystal of a larger size. Its hue ranges from a soft to a whitish pink.

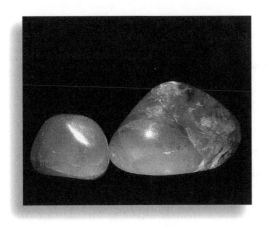

Rose Quartz essence

Rose Quartz essence dissolves negativity through gentle love and strengthens self-love. It introduces a soft, calm, loving vibration into chaotic situations and it teaches understanding of music, the arts, beauty and creativity. It is well suited for balancing, clearing and healing the emotional body. Rose Quartz essence sustains cardiac rhythm and brings joy, laughter and love into one's life. It aids the process of healing.

Affirmation:
I open my heart to the beauty of life.

Corresponding orchid: Heart Orchid

Crystal system:	Trigonal
Hardness:	9.0
Chemical formula:	Al_2O_3
Composition:	Aluminium oxide
Transparency:	Transparent to opaque
Colour:	Red
Sign of the zodiac:	Leo, Cancer, Scorpio, Sagittarius
Element:	Fire
Chakras:	Base, heart

▶ Ruby takes its name from its colour (Latin: *ruber* = red), which comes from traces of chromium. Inclusions of the mineral rutile sometimes give the effect of a glowing cat's eye or a six-pointed star. Polishing gives rubies the same radiance as diamonds.

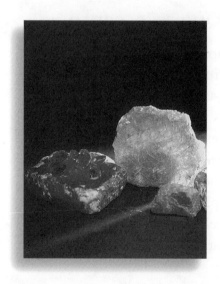

Ruby essence

Ruby essence stimulates and stabilises the base and heart chakras. It activates vital energy, invigorates the heart and achieves balance. It stimulates self-love and love for others. Physical love and mental love flow together in a harmonious way.

The fiery energy of Ruby essence gives you the courage to live your own truth, and emotional blockages are then able to dissolve.

Affirmation:
I live what I truly am.

Corresponding flower essence: Victoria Regia

RUTILATED QUARTZ

Crystal system:	Trigonal
Hardness:	6.0–7.0
Chemical formula:	$SiO_2 + TiO_2$
Composition:	Silica with titanium oxide
Transparency:	Transparent
Colour:	Colourless to smoky brown
Sign of the zodiac:	Gemini, Taurus
Element:	Fire
Chakras:	All

▶ Clear quartz and smoky quartz with inclusions of the mineral rutile (titanium oxide) grow in hexagonal prisms and are colourless or light to dark brown with yellow, golden, brownish or reddish rutile needles.

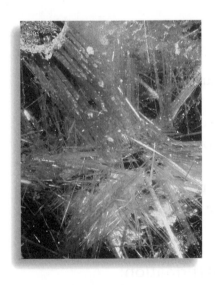

Rutilated Quartz essence

This essence helps us discover the root of our problems. The rutile needles often look like sunbeams and just like them they shine light into the dark recesses of the soul so that realisation dawns. In dreams and journeys to the higher realms, too, Rutilated Quartz essence lends greater clarity and strengthens one's capacity to remember.

The solar plexus, the place where we experience our feelings, is strengthened, emotions are felt more clearly and oppressive feelings can be eliminated.

Affirmation:
Radiant thoughts surge through me.

Corresponding orchid: Sun Orchid

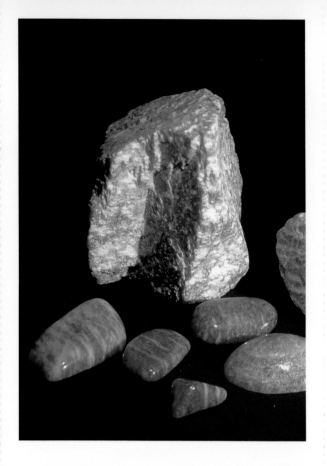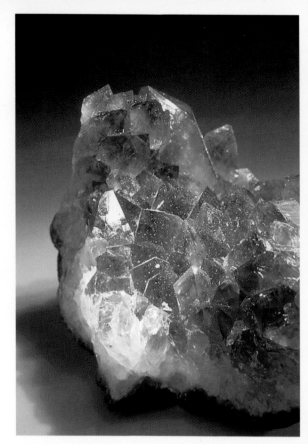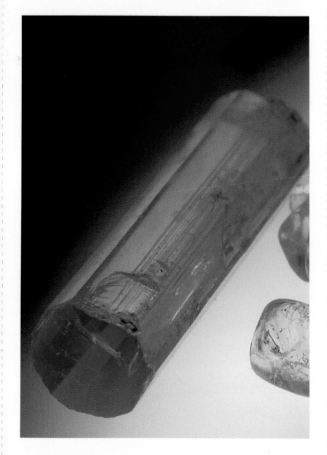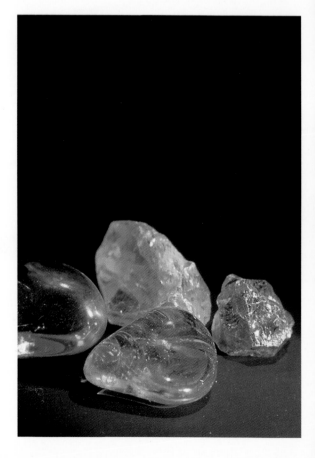

Amethyst

Amethyst is a gemstone of either a pale- or dark-purple colour with well formed tips. Sometimes it grows in light-purple groups or in the shape of a sceptre.

Affirmation:
I am filled with light and love.

Corresponding orchid:
Psyche Orchid

Amazonite

Amazonite is an opaque, green to bluish-green feldspar. Its name derives from the Amazon river.

Affirmation:
I feel well within the flow of life.

Corresponding orchid:
Deva Orchid

Citrine

Most citrines are actually heat-treated amethysts or smoky quartzes. At 450°C the colour of an amethyst changes to light yellow and at 550–560°C it changes from dark yellow to reddish brown. Smoky quartz becomes the colour of citrine at 300–400°C. Natural citrines are rather pale yellow and much more rare.

Affirmation:
Joy surges through me and opens all doors.

Corresponding orchid:
Chocolate Orchid

Aquamarine

Aquamarine is a soft, transparent light blue to blue-green. It grows as hexagonal column-shaped prisms.

Affirmation:
I can express my feelings in a free and loving way.

Corresponding essence:
Amazonas

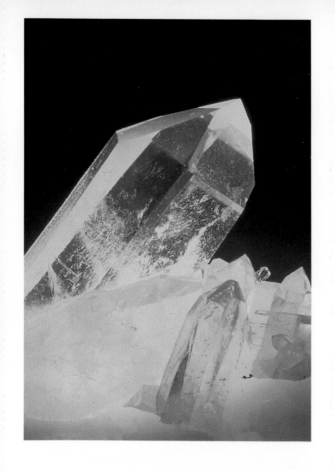 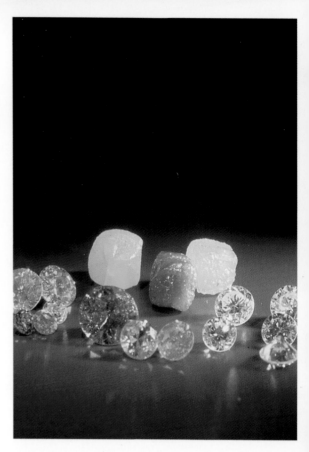

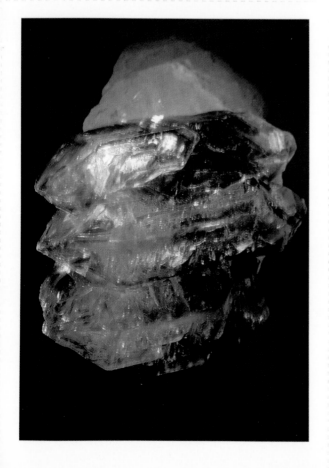 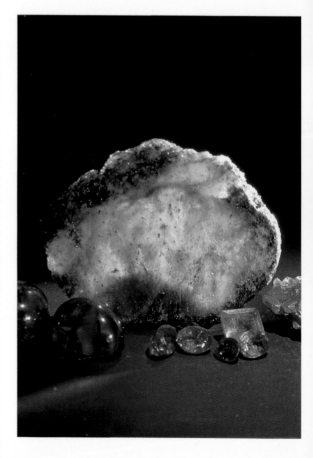

Diamond

The diamond derives its name from its hardness (Greek: *adamas* = invincible). The carbon of which it is composed is the hardest matter known. It may be colourless or can appear in a variety of colours such as yellow, brown, blue, pink and black. Due to its sparkle and refraction it is seen as the epitome of all gemstones. It grows in various shapes such as octahedra and cubes.

Affirmation:
I love myself and others, even though I recognise our weaknesses.

Corresponding orchid:
Channelling Orchid

Clear Quartz

Clear quartz grows in hexagonal prisms. Its name derives from the Greek *krystallos* (ice) because of its transparency. The crown chakra can be stimulated and opened with its help, thereby improving your connection with your Higher Self, provided that you are willing to accept your inner guidance.

Affirmation:
My Higher Self is my guide.

Corresponding orchid:
Higher Self Orchid

Emerald

Emerald grows in stem-shaped hexagonal prisms and gets its colour from chromium or vanadium. Its typical magnificent green varies from transparent to opaque. The tropical emerald with its inner six-pointed star is a renowned variety that comes from Colombia, where the indigenous peoples value it as a special stone for healing.

Affirmation:
Love dissolves all fear.

Corresponding Orchid:
Venus Orchid

Elestial Quartz
Quartz squelette

Elestial quartz is usually light to dark brown, similar to smoky quartz. It often ends in one point only; sometimes it has several points which are flattened and look like they have been compressed.

Affirmation:
I set free my pent-up energies and emotions, and I open myself up to new experiences.

Corresponding orchid:
Aggression Orchid

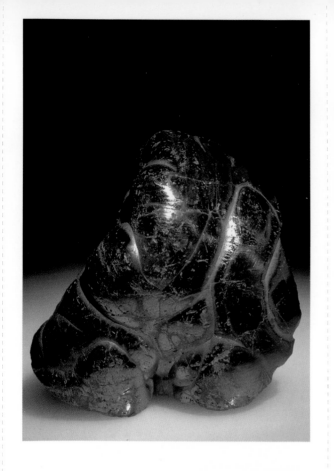

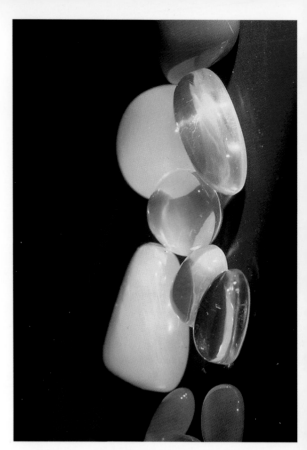

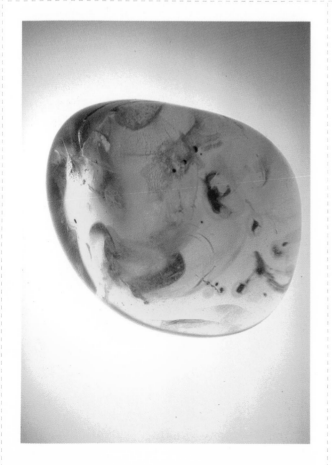

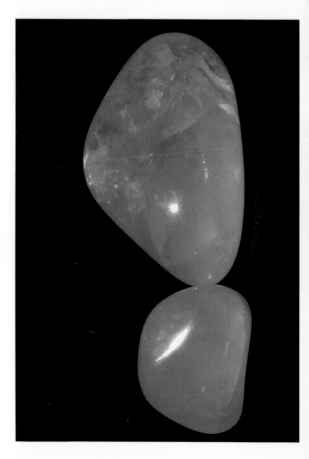

Moonstone

Moonstone is a colourless, yellow, pale blue, pink or orange feldspar. It has a bluish, pearly sheen.

Affirmation:
I give attention to my feelings and accept them, and I have a deeper understanding of others.

Corresponding orchid:
Inspiration Orchid

Haematite

Haematite grows mostly in kidney-shaped lumps or in slabs of crystal. The native North Americans utilise these haematite lumps as magic stones. Although it appears black with a silvery sheen, it is actually red. When the stone is cut, the cooling water is dyed blood red — whence its name (Greek: *haima* = blood); in some languages it is also known as 'bloodstone'.

Affirmation:
The abundance of life stimulates me.

Corresponding orchid:
Horn of Plenty Orchid

Rose Quartz

Rose quartz grows in various micro-crystalline forms, more rarely as a crystal of a larger size. Its hue ranges from a soft to a whitish pink.

Affirmation:
I open my heart to the beauty of life.

Corresponding orchid:
Heart Orchid

Olivine
Peridot — Chrysolite

Olivine is usually yellow–green, olive green (whence its name) or brownish and it grows in short rhombic prisms. It is also called peridot or chrysolite.

Affirmation:
My joy radiates outwards to everything around me.

Corresponding orchid:
Fun Orchid

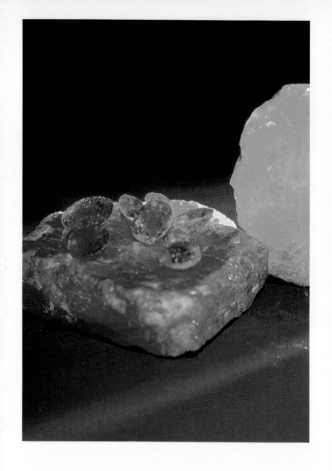 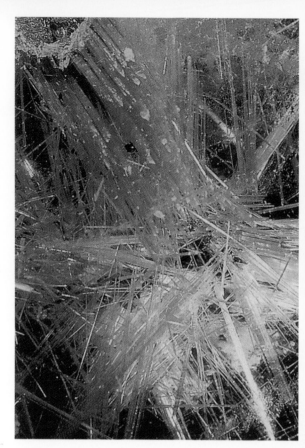

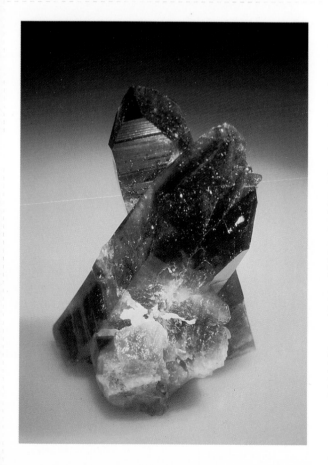 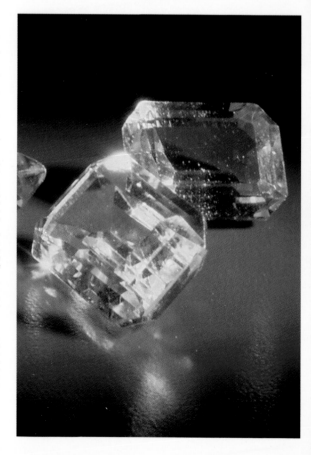

Rutilated Quartz

Clear quartz and smoky quartz with inclusions of the mineral rutile (titanium oxide) grow in hexagonal prisms and are colourless or light to dark brown with yellow, golden, brownish or reddish rutile needles.

Affirmation:
Radiant thoughts surge through me.

Corresponding orchid:
Sun Orchid

Ruby

Ruby takes its name from its colour (Latin: *ruber* = red), which comes from traces of chromium. Inclusions of the mineral rutile sometimes give the effect of a glowing cat's eye or a six-pointed star. Polishing gives rubies the same radiance as diamonds.

Affirmation:
I live what I truly am.

Corresponding flower essence:
Victoria Regia

Topaz

The golden yellow to orange topaz grows in prismatic crystals. It also occurs in colourless form or in shades of reddish brown, pinkish red, light blue and pale green. Sherry yellow topazes change their colour under the effect of heat, and blue ones are often irradiated in order to intensify their hue. Here we are dealing with the natural, sherry yellow topaz.

Affirmation:
I allow my feelings to come out and I create joy in my life.

Corresponding orchid:
Colour Orchid

Smoky Quartz

Smoky quartz is so called because of its smoky, light to dark brown colour. Sometimes it has inclusions of rutile and it mostly grows in crystal form.

Affirmation:
With every experience I come to know myself better.

Corresponding orchid:
Past Life Orchid

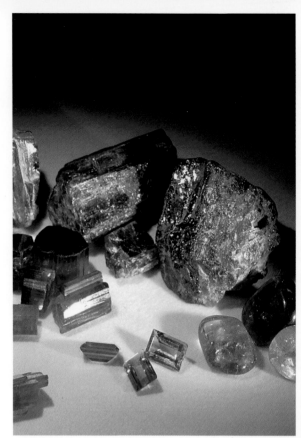

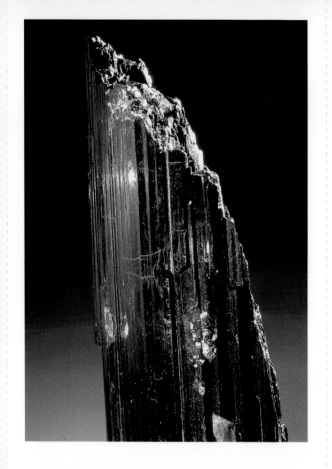

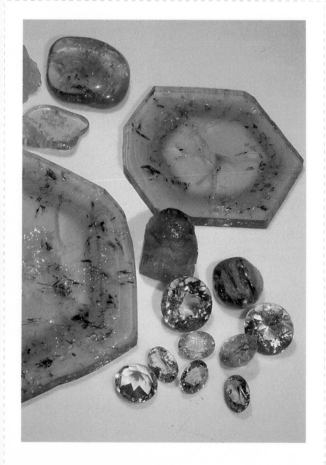

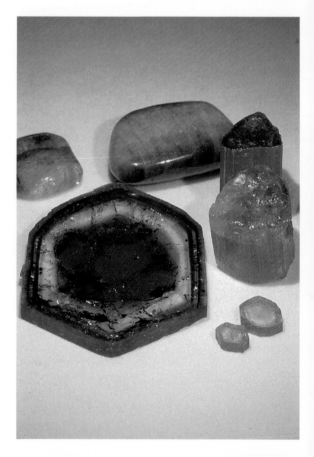

Tourmaline blue
Indicolite

Blue Tourmaline occurs in all shades of
blue. It grows in long rods of varying
thicknesses. Indicolite is rarer than black,
rose or green tourmaline.

Affirmation:
*By expressing my problems I feel light
and free.*

Corresponding orchid:
Angel Orchid

Tourmaline black
Schörl

Black Tourmaline, also known as schörl,
grows in long rods of various thicknesses.
It is opaque and vertically striated.

Affirmation:
*My guardian angel guides me safely
through the day.*

Corresponding orchid:
Angel of Protection Orchid

Tourmaline water melon
Rubellite

The watermelon tourmaline is of unusual
beauty. It grows mainly in long rods.
With its leafy green edge and pinkish red
centre it resembles a slice of watermelon.

Affirmation:
*Filled with love, I release my burdens
and am bathed in divine love.*

Corresponding orchid:
Co-ordination Orchid

Tourmaline rose
Rubellite

Rubellite grows mostly in long rods.
It appears in many different hues from pink
to red, sometimes with a light tinge of
purple. Rose Tourmaline with its more
recent history is particularly beneficial for
our present hectic and problematic age.

Affirmation:
*Filled with love, I open my heart, and
acknowledge and accept myself and others.*

Corresponding orchid:
Love Orchid

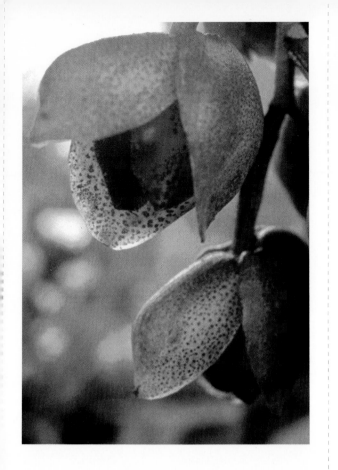
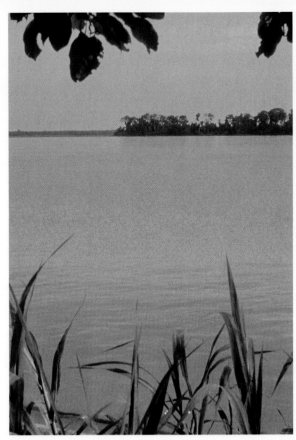
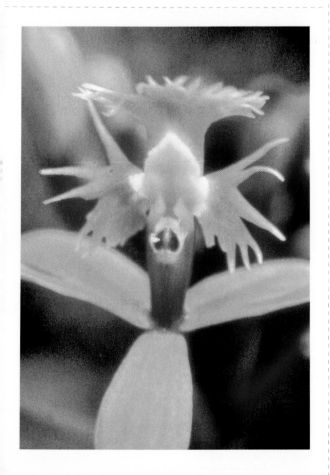
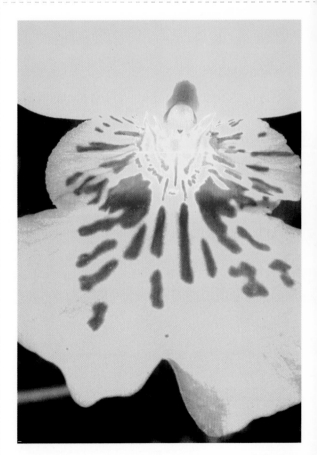

Amazonas

The Amazon flows through a forest region which, due to the multitude of species of its local flora and fauna, can be said to be the most important energetic area of the Earth.

Affirmation:
*I connect with the energetic centre
of the Earth.
I allow my energies to flow freely.*

Corresponding gem:
Aquamarine

Aggression Orchid
Acineta superba

Acineta superba has pleated leaves which grow vertically from the base of the bud; it reaches a height of up to half a metre. Its big white buds open up into red-spotted flowers that look like big open mouths with teeth and black tongues. The flower stalks hang down from the plant. This orchid has a spicy smell.

Affirmation:
*I acknowledge my aggression
and I live my sexuality.*

Corresponding gem:
Elestial Quartz

Angel of Protection Orchid
Miltonia phalaenopsis

This orchid is distinguished by its fine and delicate appearance. Its light green, slender leaves grow like tufts of grass from which the peduncles shoot out bearing usually two or three flowers. On the white blooms that resemble pansies, the contours of a figure in yellow, purple and orange-reddish hues can be made out.

Affirmation:
*My guardian angel realigns me
with my original trust.*

Corresponding gem:
Black Tourmaline

Angel Orchid
Epidendrum secundum

This essence is produced in the High Andes at a sacred place of the Chipcha Indians called Cucunuba (which means 'near the clouds'). In this variety of orchid we find flowers of all colours (red, orange, yellow, pink, blue, white, light purple).
The orchid used for the essence is of a light purple colour, which together with the white flower represents the highest level of energy.

Affirmation:
*I am light and I make contact
with the angels.*

Corresponding gem:
Blue Tourmaline

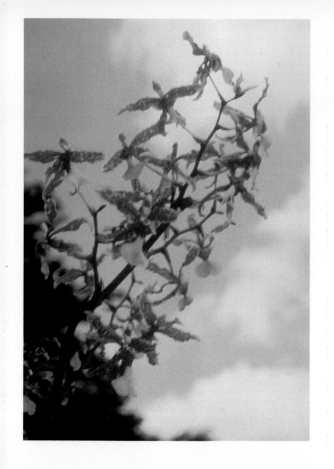
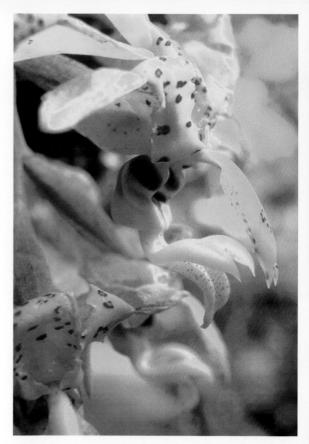
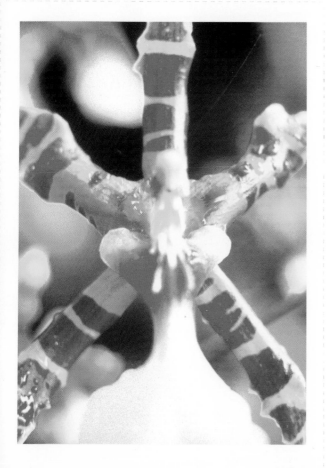
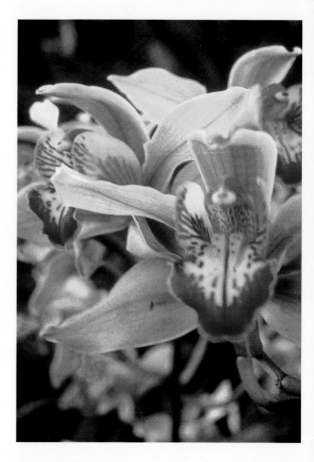

Chocolate Orchid
Stanhopea wardii

This orchid really deserves its name, as it has the sweet fragrance of the most delicate chocolate. The leaves, separate from one another, shoot out and upwards from thick buds. The flowers, not very numerous on the hanging clusters, are brownish-beige and of a very intricate structure.

Affirmation:
*I love myself. I savour what
I am, here and now.*

Corresponding gem:
Citrine

Channeling Orchid
Oncidium incurvum

This orchid has long, sword-shaped leaves out of the centre of which shoot metre-long clusters with a multitude of blossoms that all open at the same time. These small flowers are shaped like angels with white helmets.

Affirmation:
*The light is in me.
I listen to my inner voice.*

Corresponding gem:
Diamond

Co-ordination Orchid
Cymbidium lowianum

The Cymbidia belong to the variety of orchid most familiar to people, as their profusion of blooms makes them very popular as decorative plants. Their leaves are long and sword-shaped and their flowers appear mostly in winter in greenish, yellow, white and red combinations.

Affirmation:
*My consciousness expresses itself
through each cell of my body.
As within, so without.
I heal myself.*

Corresponding gem:
Watermelon Tourmaline

Colour Orchid
Miltonia clowesii

This orchid, which grows on trees, has long, sword-shaped leaves. Its long, loose flower clusters bear a multitude of blooms. These resemble small colourful angels with brownish wings, yellow faces, white dresses and haloes of lilac light around their heads.

Affirmation:
*I recognise the love that the Earth gives me.
I let the rainbow of my joy and feelings
shine.*

Corresponding gem:
Topaz

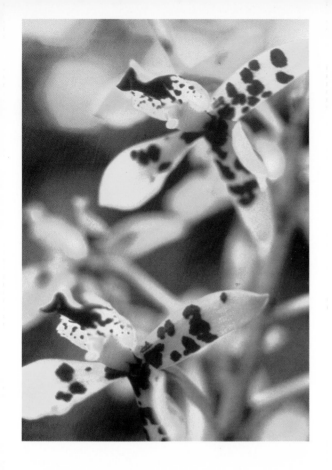
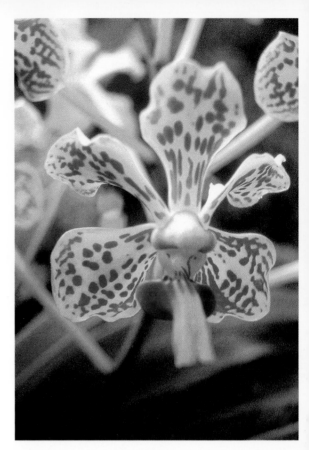
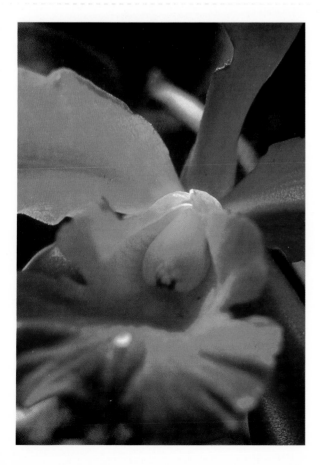
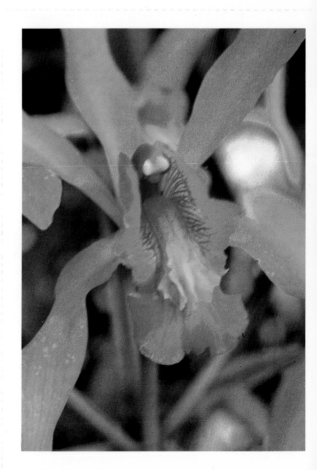

Fun Orchid
Vanda tricolor

This orchid has long leaves that grow symmetrically up the stem on opposite sides. It reaches a size of one to one-and-a-half metres, and its flowers jut out in clusters from the base of the upper leaves, resembling happy little angels.

Affirmation:
My joie de vivre makes me light-hearted. I laugh with the angels.

Corresponding gem:
Olivine

Deva Orchid
Epidendrum prismatocarpum

This orchid can be recognised by its root-like growths massed together on the rhizome and its large, textured, egg-shaped leaves, flattened at their tips and spiralling up the stalk. The flowers appear in large numbers along the vertical main stem on which they too grow in a spiral. The flowers look like green angels with white head-dresses.

Affirmation:
I open my heart to the message of the flowers.

Corresponding gem:
Amazonite

Higher Self Orchid
Laeliocattleya anceps clara

This orchid, which is found in the Brazilian part of Amazonia, usually has two leaves. Its flower stalk, about a metre tall, carries its flowers at its tip. The orchid used for the essence is a bright lilac colour with a yellow centre.

Affirmation:
I am the expression of my Higher Self. I am open and my field of vision is becoming wider.

Corresponding gem:
Clear Quartz

Heart Orchid
Laeliocattleya hybride

The Laeliocattleyae occur mainly in the Brazilian part of Amazonia and over the course of time they have produced a great number of different varieties.

Affirmation:
I open my heart to infinite love.

Corresponding gem:
Rose Quartz

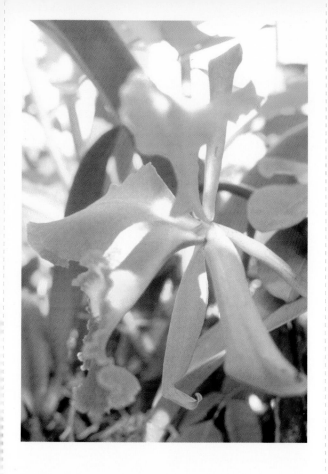
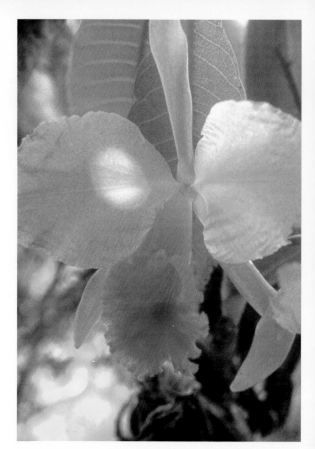
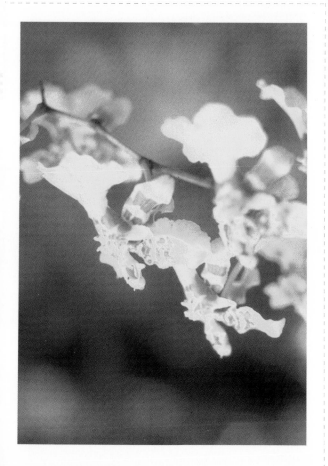
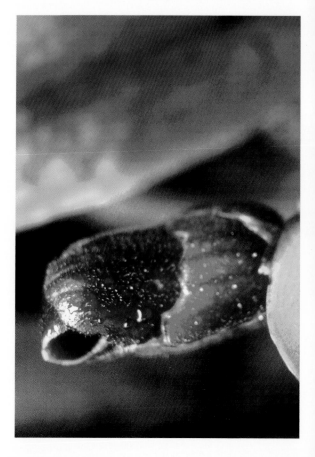

Inspiration Orchid
Cattleya trianae

Cattleya trianae is one of the best known orchids of the Cattleya family. There are many varieties in different colours. The Cattleya used here is dark lilac with a yellow centre. Cattleya trianae is the emblem of Colombia.

Affirmation:
I connect with divine love, and I receive it into myself.

Corresponding gem:
Moonstone

Horn of Plenty Orchid
Cattleya warscewiczii

A characteristic of Cattleya warscewiczii, along with other varieties of Cattleya, is its centre labellum which grows in a flourish and looks like a horn of plenty.

Affirmation:
The love of the universe flows through me into the earth.

Corresponding gem:
Haematite

Past Life Orchid
Paphiopedilum harrysianum

This orchid has long leaves with rounded tips that grow in the shape of a fan; from their centre springs a single peduncle. For the production of this essence, only buds which have just opened are used. They are ovate and hollow.

Affirmation:
All knowledge is within me and shows me the way.

Corresponding gem:
Smoky Quartz

Love Orchid
Oncidium abortivum

This orchid which grows exclusively on trees is one of the best known Oncidia. Its leaves are arranged lengthways. Its delicate yellow flowers shoot out from the axils in large numbers on long panicles. Each flower is shaped like a little angel with a three-cornered hat and a heart chakra which has a special mark.

Affirmation:
I let love flow through me. I heal myself and I heal others.

Corresponding gem:
Rose Tourmaline

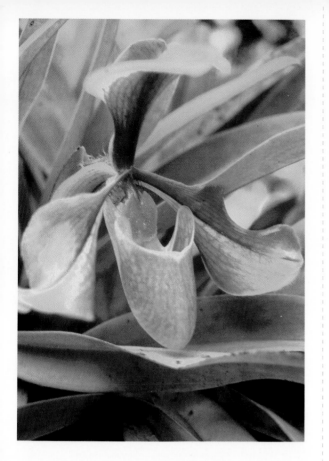 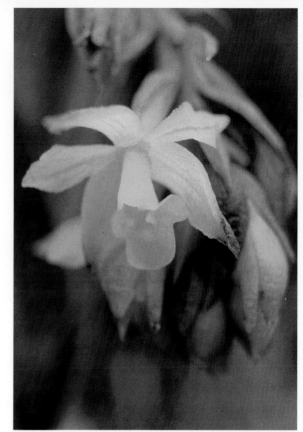

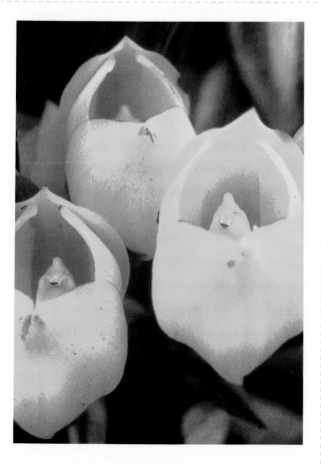 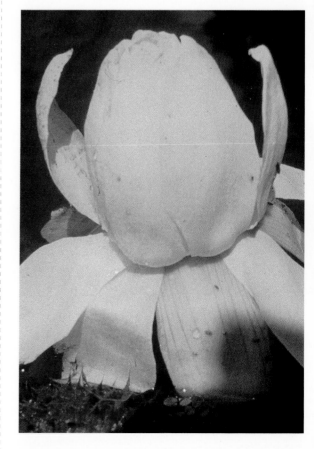

Sun Orchid
Epidendrum chioneum

This terrestrial orchid, which reaches a
height of twenty to thirty-five centimetres, is
a species that grows on the mountain peaks
of Chingaza, an area sacred to the Indians.
It grows vertically from the ground.

Affirmation:
The sun shines within me.
The cosmos and I are one.

Corresponding gem:
Rutilated Quartz

Psyche Orchid
Paphiopedilum insigne

The Paphiopedilum genus constitutes one of
the best known varieties of orchid.
Their long leaves rounded off at the tips
produce one single flower or several
separate flowers with a characteristic
slipper-shaped labellum.

Affirmation:
I am.
I am part of the divine plan.
I am.

Corresponding gem:
Amethyst

Victoria Regia Orchid
Victoria amazonica

Victoria Regia belongs to the family of
Nymphaeaceae and is the largest kind of
water lily found in the world.
Its leaves can grow to a diameter of two
metres or more, while its white flowers in
comparison are rather small (20-30 cm).
It floats on the surface
of the lakes and lagoons of Amazonia.

Affirmation:
My energies flow freely and lightly.
I have trust and I let go.

Corresponding gem:
Ruby

Venus Orchid
Anguloa cliftonii

Long, fan-shaped, linear leaves grow out of
its small, stocky bud and the plant grows up
to half a metre in height. The yellow or
sometimes white flowers appear in ones or
twos at the bottom of the leaf stalk.
The shape of the flower resembles
the female sex organ.

Affirmation:
I accept the feminine part of myself.
I am gentleness and love.

Corresponding gem:
Emerald

SMOKY QUARTZ

Crystal system:	Trigonal
Hardness:	7.0
Chemical formula:	SiO_2
Composition:	Silica
Transparency:	Transparent to opaque
Colour:	Light brown, dark brown
Sign of the zodiac:	Capricorn, Sagittarius
Element:	Water
Chakras:	Base, sacral, solar plexus

▶ Smoky quartz is so called because of its smoky, light to dark brown colour. Sometimes it has inclusions of rutile and it mostly grows in crystal form.

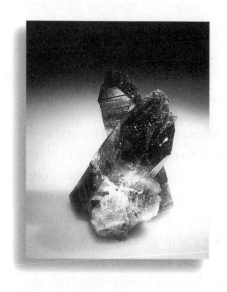

Smoky Quartz essence

Smoky Quartz essence provides the stability necessary to open up to new experiences and also to look at and accept our own shadow side and experiences from past lifetimes. We recognise that learning processes are necessary, although they sometimes hurt. Feelings are tidied up and we learn to accept ourself just as we are. In this way Smoky Quartz essence helps to balance body and soul.

Affirmation:
With every experience I come to know myself better.

Corresponding orchid: Past Life Orchid

TOPAZ

Crystal system:	Orthorhombic
Hardness:	8.0
Chemical formula:	$Al_2(SiO_4)(F,OH)_2$
Composition:	Aluminium fluorosilicate
Transparency:	Transparent
Colour:	Golden yellow to orange
Sign of the zodiac:	Sagittarius, Leo, Pisces
Element:	Air
Chakras:	Solar plexus, third eye

▶ The golden yellow to orange topaz grows in prismatic crystals. It also occurs in colourless form or in shades of reddish brown, pinkish red, light blue and pale green. Sherry yellow topazes change their colour under the effect of heat, and blue ones are often irradiated in order to intensify their hue. Here we are dealing with the natural, sherry yellow topaz.

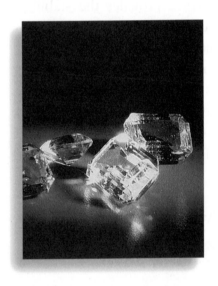

Topaz essence

Topaz essence replaces negativity with joy and love. It allows our feelings to rise from the solar plexus to the third eye: from the internal sun, the world of emotions, onto the level of consciousness. Our consciousness is flooded with an energy similar to the sun's and we become more aware of our hidden and suppressed feelings. The world appears more colourful and alive. Topaz essence stimulates the digestive and detoxifying organs of the body and tones and balances the nervous system and solar plexus.

Affirmation:
I allow my feelings to come out and I create joy in my life.

Corresponding orchid: Colour Orchid

black TOURMALINE
— Schorl —

Crystal system:	Trigonal
Hardness:	7.0–7.5
Chemical formula:	$NaFe_3(Al,Fe^{3+})_6((OH)_4/(BO_3)_3/Si_6O_{18})$
Composition:	Complex borosilicate
Transparency:	Opaque
Colour:	Black
Sign of the zodiac:	Capricorn
Element:	Earth
Chakras:	Base, feet

▶ Black Tourmaline, also known as schorl, grows in long rods of various thicknesses. It is opaque and vertically striated.

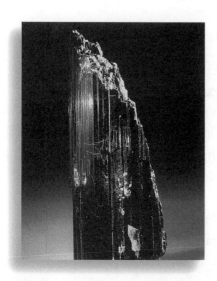

Black Tourmaline essence

This essence strengthens one's connection with the earth and is particularly suitable for people who do not live in the here and now. It has a detoxifying effect on kidneys and intestines. It is beneficial in cases of over-exposure to radiation from computers, electric appliances and screens, eliminating negative vibrations in body and mind. In addition it stimulates the immune system. It brings to light shadow areas which can then be accepted.

Affirmation:
My guardian angel guides me safely through the day.

Corresponding orchid: Angel of Protection Orchid

TOURMALINE blue
— *Indicolite* —

Crystal system:	Trigonal
Hardness:	7.0–7.5
Chemical formula:	$(Na, Li, Ca)(Mn, Mg, Fe, Al, Ti, Cr)_9 (OH, F)_4/(Bo_3)_3/Si_6O_{18})$
Composition:	Complex borosilicate
Transparency:	Transparent to opaque
Colour:	All shades of blue
Sign of the zodiac:	Taurus
Element:	Water
Chakras:	Solar plexus, throat, third eye

▶ Blue Tourmaline occurs in all shades of blue. It grows in long rods of varying thicknesses. Indicolite is rarer than black, rose or green tourmaline.

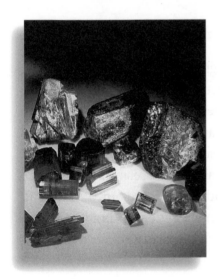

Blue Tourmaline essence

Blue Tourmaline essence allows emotions bottled up in the solar plexus to surface and be expressed verbally. It acts on the thyroid gland and strengthens the lungs. It also awakens the feminine, an aspect that is often repressed in humans. It promotes deep sleep, relieves depression and counteracts stress.

Blue Tourmaline essence increases sensitivity to the refined vibrations of angels.

Affirmation:
By expressing my problems I feel light and free.

Corresponding orchid: Angel Orchid

rose TOURMALINE
— Rubellite —

Crystal system:	Trigonal
Hardness:	7.0–7.5
Chemical formula:	$(Na, Li, Ca)(Mn, Mg, Fe, Al, Ti, Cr)_9 (OH, F)_4/(Bo_3)_3/Si_6O_{18})$
Composition:	Complex borosilicate
Transparency:	Transparent to opaque
Colour:	Pink to red
Sign of the zodiac:	Sagittarius, Scorpio
Element:	Water
Chakras:	Sacral, heart, solar plexus

▶ Rubellite grows mostly in long rods. It appears in many different hues from pink to red, sometimes with a light tinge of purple. Rose Tourmaline with its more recent history is particularly beneficial for our present hectic and problematic age.

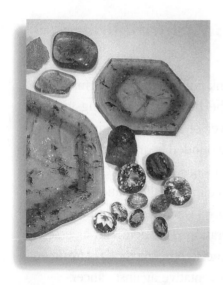

Rose Tourmaline essence

This essence frees the heart area of blockages that have arisen from negative experiences in the past. It heals old wounds and restores lightness and fun. Blockages of the heart that are beginning to manifest on the physical level are dissolved by the action of the lithium contained in Tourmaline. Prejudices evaporate and are replaced by higher knowledge; this new start gives rise to loving actions which come from the heart. Raised self-esteem gears you up to new deeds.

Affirmation:
Filled with love, I open my heart, and acknowledge and accept myself and others.

Corresponding orchid: Love Orchid

T watermelon OURMALINE

Crystal system:	Trigonal
Hardness:	7.0–7.5
Chemical formula:	$(Na, Li, Ca) (Mn, Mg, Fe, Al, Ti, Cr)_9 ((OH, F)_4/(Bo_3)_3/Si_6O_{18})$
Composition:	Complex borosilicate
Transparency:	Transparent to opaque
Colour:	Greenish pink
Sign of the zodiac:	Virgo, Gemini
Element:	Water
Chakras:	Sacral, heart, solar plexus

▶ The watermelon tourmaline is of unusual beauty. It grows mainly in long rods. With its leafy green edge and pinkish red centre it resembles a slice of watermelon.

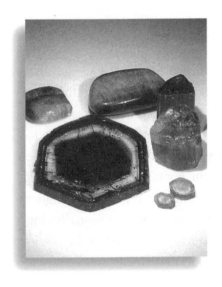

Watermelon Tourmaline essence

The green and pink colours of this tourmaline are associated with the heart. The soothing green is good for the power of self-healing, and the pink helps to heal the wounded heart, to open it up and to dissolve old blockages. Disturbances in the soul sometimes cause cellular malformation. Using the essence and wearing a watermelon tourmaline assist in cellular regeneration. This gem and its essence are a valuable adjunct to other methods of treatment, especially as a preventative against cancer.

Affirmation:
Filled with love, I release my burdens and am bathed in divine love.

Corresponding orchid: Co-ordination Orchid

the ORCHIDS and their ESSENCES

The Orchids

In Europe, including the Mediterranean basin, a total of 264 different kinds of orchid are found. But within the land area of Colombia alone, where the world's greatest concentration of flora and fauna species exists, four thousand different varieties of orchid have been recorded.

Orchids belong to the most recent species in the evolution of the plant kingdom. With some 25–35,000 different kinds existing throughout the world, orchids have attained a huge variety of forms — even some that imitate insects, organs and symbols. Particularly astonishing are those that look like angels or other tiny beings! This magnificent imagery with its abundance of shapes and colours is the hallmark of orchids' high-level energetic specialisation.

The orchids of Europe and the Mediterranean region are, just like other plants and flowers, rooted in the earth and therefore intimately linked with it. By analogy, on an energetic level they are directly connected with the human body: they work on our seven body chakras and affect us mainly on the astral level. Due to the particular distribution of light in Amazonia many species of orchid there have developed roots that are no longer tied to the soil. They only have support roots and are found in the treetops, on the 'top floor' of the humid rainforest. Here, at a height of 25–35 metres, they lead, as do other epiphytes, a life that is independent of the tree they live in.

What does it imply, that these plants no longer live in direct contact with the earth? From an energetic point of view, it means that their actions go beyond the physical level. Just as they grow in the treetops which, in energetic terms, represent the astral body, so does their effect begin in the astral body and from there extends to the other subtle bodies.

Orchids and the Higher Chakras

Above the seven chakras linked with the physical body there are five more which we call the higher chakras. We have already mentioned them in relation to gemstones. The eighth chakra is linked with the right hemisphere of the brain, that of intuitive thinking. This is the point, situated above the seventh chakra, where the soul is connected to the monad (in Greek: unity). The ninth chakra corresponds to the third eye and the left brain, which is concerned with logical thinking. The tenth chakra is related to creativity and higher aspiration. The eleventh chakra is the centre which is linked to each cell nucleus of our physical body. It is responsible for their formation. The twelfth chakra is directly linked to the divine Source.

Orchids that grow as epiphytes work on the higher chakras. They therefore represent contact of the human being and the Earth with the cosmos and the various realms of the invisible world. They can be seen as the highest developmental level of the plant kingdom.

The Orchid Essences

Due to their high vibratory frequency the collection of orchid essences provides, to our knowledge, the most subtle energies of all essences available. Gemstones come from the entrails of the earth and so are linked with the physical level. In fact we know that gem essences work mainly on the physical body. There is, however, a subtle transition between gem essences and flower essences. Opaque stones, for example black tourmaline or obsidian, work predominantly on the physical aspect of the human body. Clear, transparent stones, such as quartz or diamond, influence both the physical aspect of the body and the spiritual or soul level.

Flowers, bushes and trees are connected by their roots to the earth and thus to the physical realm. This is why flower essences affect the various body chakras. In general, however, their role in the physical realm is much less important than that of the gemstone essences. Although the plants are still linked to the earth, they grow up vertically above its surface, in the same way that human beings stand upright on the ground. Most of their energy, though, is concentrated in their upper part, the flower, which contains the reproductive organs. Energetically their effect goes beyond the boundary formed by the skin, and penetrates the subtle regions of the body.

There exists within the plant kingdom a hierarchy of evolution. In this respect we could refer to algae or poisonous plants as of a 'lower' nature. For the most part, their action takes place on a low energy level. Then come the plants that affect the lower chakras, such as basil (*Basilicum officinalis*) which works on the sacral chakra or clematis (*Clematis vitalba*) which stimulates the feet. Plants which affect the solar plexus and heart are, for example, the sunflower (*Helianthus annuus*) (solar plexus) or holly (*Ilex aquifolium*) (heart chakra). Finally we come to the astral and spiritual realms. We call flowers related to these 'higher plants', for example sage (*Salvia officinalis*) or passion flower (*Passionaria hybride*). They stimulate the higher chakras of the body.

Between the flower and orchid essences we can place so-called 'transition flowers' whose vibrations affect the astral body on a higher level. Here we find flowers such as the lotus (*Nelumbo nucifera*) or Victoria Regia (*Victoria amazonica*). The family of the *Orchidaceae*, the orchids, represents the most recent development in the evolution of plants, just as humankind represents the highest level of specialisation in mammals alongside dolphins and whales.

The orchids of Amazonia are mostly so-called epiphytes. They live on trees and no longer have any direct contact with the earth. They live, energetically speaking, above the astral body, which is represented by the tree. These orchids vibrate in the higher realms and represent the connection between the cosmos, human beings and Earth. They help us get in contact with various levels of the cosmic love of the angels and allow us to pass on this experience of love to the Earth; in so doing they help us to heal ourselves and the whole planet.

It is not by chance that right now, at the start of the Age of Aquarius, we are becoming aware of the orchid essences. As more and more people develop spiritually, some of them are going to respond to orchid essences, which accelerate this very process of evolution. The first of these essences were produced in 1990. Due to the large number of orchids we are still just at the beginning of a vast research project, but in this task, too, we will evolve, just like our planet.

The following descriptions are direct messages received from the devas of the orchids during the production of the essences.

Energy levels

Orchid essences	higher chakras; angel realm
Higher flower essences	upper body chakras
Central flower essences	heart chakra, solar plexus
Lower flower essences	lower body chakras
Higher gem essences	physical and psycho-spiritual level
Lower gem essences	physical level

We assume, however, that the essences have an even greater range of effects and that in due course we will gain more information. Before applying the essences it is recommended that you check them out by means of one of the intuitive tests described earlier and that you use them with full awareness of your responsibility. Their high vibratory frequencies can trigger powerful energies in human beings (particularly Aggression Orchid and Victoria Regia).

In our work since 1990 we have been able to establish that in certain cases a better energy impact is achieved by *external application* of the orchid essences.

Making Orchid Essences

As orchids are especially highly developed plants it is absolutely necessary to produce these essences in a way which does not harm the plant. Unlike the gem essences, it is not possible to produce your own orchid essences.

In collaboration with researchers in Paris, Andreas Korte has developed a technique which avoids the actual picking of the flowers. Only their energetic body is used. Essences made by this method have proved more powerful than those produced on the same day following the conventional method, because the plants are not traumatised by cutting; they retain their energy intact and this is transmitted into the essence.

The crystal method

This method combines flowers and crystals, the highest expressions of the plant and mineral kingdoms respectively, in order to obtain essences. For this, a quartz crystal geode which has been prepared in a certain way is used.

Apart from this the production of the flower essences does not differ from the classical method devised by Dr Edward Bach. We need:

▶ a large amount of the best quality of the relevant species of flower;

▶ a perfectly protected place, far from any disturbances such as streets, industry, electric wires or other sources of pollution;

▶ auspicious timing in relation to the phases of the moon (full moon, waxing moon);

▶ a blue and sunny sky;

▶ personal well-being in order to avoid our vibrations adversely affecting the production process.

When all these conditions have been met, and we have found a suitable place, we have to get into perfect harmony with the plants. For Andreas Korte this is a crucial factor. He only produces essences when he senses the devas of the plants calling him and asking him to make an essence. In this case he begins by meditating for a while with the plants and communicating with them. Then he gets in touch with the various elemental forces to ask them for their assistance in the production process. Only then does he get in touch with the crystal geode in order to prepare it for the work at hand and to reassure himself of its cooperation. He then fills the geode with clear, pure spring water and places it within the energetic body of the flowers. Finally he senses how the devas and the crystal begin to work: the energetic body of the plants is wrung out like a moist sponge and the energies are conducted into the water via the crystal. At the end of this process, which takes several hours, he thanks the devas, the crystal and the elemental forces before mixing the mother tincture with alcohol.

This new method of producing flower essences works directly with the energetic body of the plants in order to produce a remedy that can be used to treat the energetic body of humans or other living beings. It has two distinct advantages. First, the plant is neither destroyed nor suffers in any other way, as its energetic body recharges during the night and following morning. Second, this method achieves a very high-energy essence, free of any vibrations of suffering.

DESCRIPTIONS
of the ESSENCES

▶

Note: In this book, the orchids are designated by their botanical name and the essences by mostly English names made up by the authors (for example: Aggression Orchid, *Acineta superba*).

AMAZONAS
— River Essence —

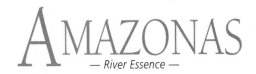

The Amazon flows through a forest region which, due to the multitude of species of its local flora and fauna, can be said to be the most important energetic area of the Earth.

Amazonas essence

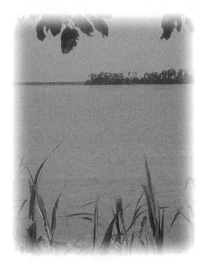

This essence, made by the crystal method, aligns us with the enormous energy of the Amazon river. It takes us to the energetic centre of the Earth.

With the help of this essence we develop an understanding of our planet and all the beings that live on it. On a physical level the Amazon river corresponds with our spine and helps our life energy flow. This essence helps us to eliminate physical blockages, which can be swept away by this mighty river. It has often proved successful in the treatment of back pain.

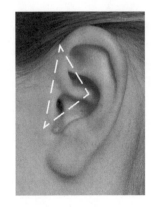

A cotton bud soaked in the essence is applied directly to the outer ear, and the fossa triangularis, which corresponds to the spinal column, is stimulated. The message of the essence is thus transmitted directly into the back via the nervous system. Both ears should be stimulated simultaneously. Very shortly afterwards the patient will feel heat in his or her back; this indicates that vital energy is beginning to circulate in a previously blocked area.

Note: It is important to test the essence beforehand

Affirmation:
I connect with the energetic centre of the Earth.
I allow my energies to flow freely.

Corresponding gem: Aquamarine

AGGRESSION ORCHID
— Acineta superba —

Acineta superba has pleated leaves which grow vertically from the base of the bud; it reaches a height of up to half a metre. Its big white buds open up into red-spotted flowers that look like big open mouths with teeth and black tongues. The flower stalks hang down from the plant. This orchid has a spicy smell.

Aggression Orchid essence

This essence has to be used with caution as it releases blockages of the first chakra — sexuality, violence and repressed aggression. It can be like an explosion that surges up from below. These energies that have been blocked in the first chakra over a long period need to be expressed so that they can be transformed. It is important that the first chakra is unblocked so that the flow of vital energy can circulate upwards in a permanent flow, and so that it can eventually connect with our higher chakras. This is the only way for us to reach a balanced state. This orchid helps us to accept repressed feelings and integrate them.

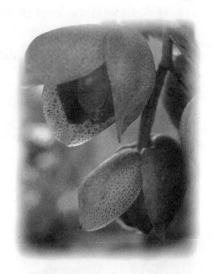

Note: This orchid has such a lot of energy that it even heated up the crystal during its production!

Affirmation:
I acknowledge my aggression and I live my sexuality.

Corresponding gem: Elestial Quartz

ANGEL ORCHID
— *Epidendrum secundum* —

This essence is produced in the High Andes at a sacred place of the Chipcha Indians called Cucunuba (which means 'near the clouds').

In this variety of orchid we find flowers of all colours (red, orange, yellow, pink, blue, white, light purple). The orchid used for the essence is of a light purple colour, which together with the white flower represents the highest level of energy.

Angel Orchid essence

This orchid allows us to enter into communication with the angels. Still rooted in the earth, it corresponds to the third eye in the human body, which is confirmed by a dot on the peduncle, a characteristic feature of this flower. First we find ourselves on the level of the base petals; then via the third eye we get in touch with a rising energy which raises our consciousness further and further until our level of vibration finally allows us to make contact with very high realms.

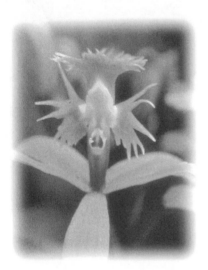

This essence makes us light and joyful. Raising vibrations, lightness and expanding consciousness are its main qualities.

Affirmation:
I am light and I make contact with the angels.

Corresponding gem: Blue Tourmaline

ANGEL of PROTECTION ORCHID
— Miltonia phalaenopsis —

This orchid is distinguished by its fine and delicate appearance. Its light green, slender leaves grow like tufts of grass from which the peduncles shoot out bearing usually two or three flowers. On the white blooms that resemble pansies the contours of a figure in yellow, purple and orange-reddish hues can be made out.

Angel of Protection Orchid essence

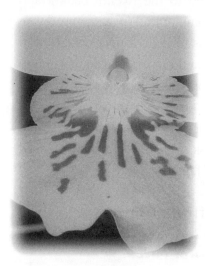

This essence puts us in contact with our guardian angel. It is suitable particularly for refined, sensitive characters who feel exposed to all kinds of hostility in difficult surroundings and who urgently require a protective shield around themselves to deflect negative vibrations. Just as the delicate figure is surrounded by a white shield, our angel protects us, and the orchid helps us to connect more easily with our angel.

Affirmation:
My guardian angel realigns me with my original trust.

Corresponding gem: Black Tourmaline

CHANNELLING ORCHID
— Oncidium incurvum —

This orchid has long, sword-shaped leaves out of the centre of which shoot metre-long clusters with a multitude of blossoms that all open at the same time. These small flowers are shaped like angels with white helmets.

Channelling Orchid essence

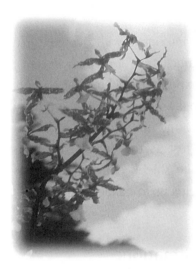

This orchid is linked to the twelfth chakra and represents direct communication with the divine source. It enables us to make direct contact with our spiritual guides and our original source and to receive messages from these in order to share them with others.

It is suitable for people who have dedicated themselves to the task of channelling and who need support in times of fatigue.

Affirmation:
The light is in me. I listen to my inner voice.

Corresponding gem: Diamond

CHOCOLATE ORCHID
— Stanhopea wardii —

This orchid really deserves its name, as it has the sweet fragrance of the most delicate chocolate. The leaves, separate from one another, shoot out and upwards from thick buds. The flowers, not very numerous on the hanging clusters, are brownish-beige and of a very intricate structure.

Chocolate Orchid essence

The shape of its wide-open flower, which gives out a delicate chocolate perfume, teaches us that the spiritual life is also something sweet and pleasurable. It is aimed at those who believe that spirituality is something strictly serious and who tend to be bitter. Everything in life is a treat if that is how we create it in our mind! This orchid essence is suitable, for example, for very rigid people with a thin and sad appearance, who think everything ought to be done according to strict rules.

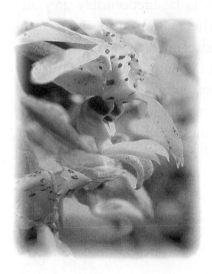

It helps us to connect with the spiritual world and truly to know what is good for us and what is not. It also helps us to understand that everything in life has its rightful place and that we should not limit ourselves.

Affirmation:
I love myself. I savour what I am, here and now.

Corresponding gem: Citrine

COLOUR ORCHID
— Miltonia clowesii —

This orchid, which grows on trees, has long, sword-shaped leaves. Its long, loose flower clusters bear a multitude of blooms. These resemble small colourful angels with brownish wings, yellow faces, white dresses and haloes of lilac light around their heads.

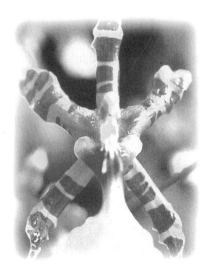

Colour Orchid essence

A closer look at this orchid shows that although it has a sad background (light to dark brown), it surges up into the colours of life (white, lilac, yellow) which appear in the foreground. It could also be called the orchid that elevates thinking. It is suited to people with a tendency towards sadness, who believe their lives to be irredeemably grey and hopeless. This orchid helps us recognise that it is uniquely the quality of our thoughts that influences our perception of the outside world. With happy and joyful thoughts, our world becomes colourful and extraordinary. The spiritual world does not want us to feel sad. On the contrary, it wants us to be fully ourselves in the joy of life, so that we can recognise the love which the Earth gives us. Finally, we learn to offer our joy and love to others.

To release us from grey thoughts and open us up to life and love are the main properties of this orchid.

Affirmation:
I recognise the love that the Earth gives me.
I let the rainbow of my joy and feelings shine.

Corresponding gem: Topaz

CO-ORDINATION ORCHID
— *Cymbidium lowianum* —

The *Cymbidia* belong to the variety of orchid most familiar to people, as their profusion of blooms makes them very popular as decorative plants. Their leaves are long and sword-shaped and their flowers appear mostly in winter in greenish, yellow, white and red combinations.

Co-ordination Orchid essence

This orchid connects us with the eleventh chakra, the centre of Co-ordination and organisation of the physical structure. The nucleus of each of our cells is directly linked to it and therefore to the cosmos as well. It represents the place of administration of the cosmic form and its laws of manifestation.

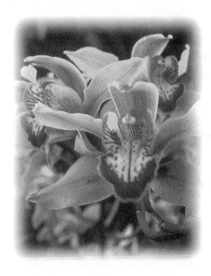

Pathological mutations of form can also be of genetic origin. This orchid helps us to allow the healing energy of the eleventh chakra circulate within us. It is a powerful energy which can be felt in the heart and the anterior part of the brain.

Affirmation:
My consciousness expresses itself through each cell of my body. As within, so without. I heal myself.

Corresponding gem: Watermelon Tourmaline

DEVA ORCHID

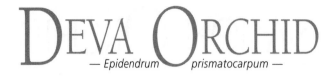

— Epidendrum prismatocarpum —

This orchid can be recognised by its root-like growths massed together on the rhizome and its large, textured, egg-shaped leaves, flattened at their tips and spiralling up the stalk. The flowers appear in large numbers along the vertical main stem on which they too grow in a spiral. The flowers look like green angels with white head-dresses.

Deva Orchid essence

This orchid puts us in touch with the natural energies of the various elements on a subtle level. It opens our consciousness to the experience of communicating with the devas of flowers and trees, the elemental forces of the mineral kingdom and the water spirits.

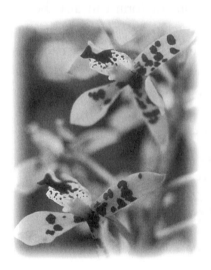

It renders us receptive, it opens us up and thus facilitates our perception. It helps us to break down the barriers that separate us from the invisible realm.

Affirmation:
I open my heart to the message of the flowers.

Corresponding gem: Amazonite

HORN OF PLENTY ORCHID
Cattleya warscewiczii —

A characteristic of *Cattleya warscewiczii*, along with other varieties of *Cattleya*, is its centre labellum which grows in a flourish and looks like a horn of plenty.

Horn of Plenty Orchid essence

Horn of Plenty Orchid essence represents the connection between the cosmos and Earth. We experience the infinite love of the universe, let it flow through us and pass it on to the earth. We have a feeling of stimulation in our feet and get in touch with the earth. This orchid essence establishes a connection between heaven, human beings and earth. It helps us to understand that everything exists in abundance, just like cosmic love, and that there are no limits. We learn how to become

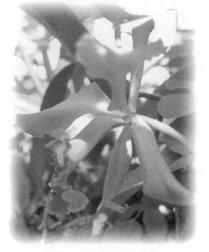

a horn of plenty, giving and receiving. In the same way we learn to accept consciously all the gifts of the universe and to pass on this love to the earth.

Affirmation:
The love of the universe flows through me into the earth.

Corresponding gem: Haematite

FUN ORCHID
— Vanda tricolor —

This orchid has long leaves that grow symmetrically up the stem on opposite sides. It reaches a size of one to one-and-a-half metres, and its flowers jut out in clusters from the base of the upper leaves, resembling happy little angels.

Fun Orchid essence

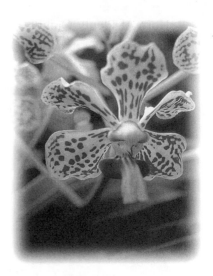

To dance with the angels is a joy. This essence increases our sense of humour and our joie de vivre. It makes us light-hearted and cheerful. It stimulates our higher chakras and helps us gain access to realms where we can look at our problems in a different light and be happy.

This orchid essence is suitable for sad, depressed people, helping them to release their inner tension. It awakens the child in us and helps us to become happy and relaxed.

Affirmation:
*My joie de vivre makes me light-hearted.
I laugh with the angels.*

Corresponding gem: Olivine

HEART ORCHID
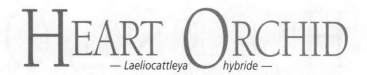
— Laeliocattleya hybride —

The *Laeliocattleyae* occur mainly in the Brazilian part of Amazonia and over the course of time they have produced a great number of different varieties.

Heart Orchid essence

This orchid essence enables us to boost our energies. Egoistic emotions on the level of the solar plexus rise to the heart chakra and turn into love. To see with the eyes of the heart and to coordinate our acts of love with the spiritual world — these are the qualities developed by this essence.

Affirmation:
I open my heart to infinite love.

Corresponding gem: Rose Quartz

HIGHER SELF ORCHID
— Laeliocattleya anceps clara —

This orchid, which is found in the Brazilian part of Amazonia, usually has two leaves. Its flower stalk, about a metre tall, carries its flowers at its tip. The orchid used for the essence is a bright lilac colour with a yellow centre.

Higher Self Orchid essence

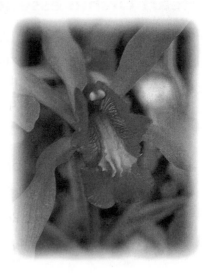

This essence connects us with our Higher Self, enhancing our ability to receive its information. It purifies and opens our higher chakras and thus enables us to receive cosmic love and let it flow through us. It stimulates us to broaden our perspective. It also increases our capacity to get in touch with the spiritual world.

Affirmation:
I am the expression of my Higher Self. I am open and my field of vision is becoming wider.

Corresponding gem: Clear Quartz

INSPIRATION ORCHID
— Cattleya trianae —

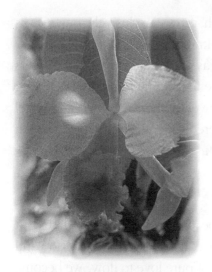

Cattleya trianae is one of the best known orchids of the *Cattleya* family. There are many varieties in different colours. The *Cattleya* used here is dark lilac with a yellow centre. *Cattleya trianae* is the emblem of Colombia.

Inspiration Orchid essence

This essence facilitates the transformation of aggressive energy into inspiration. We could compare this orchid to the iris, except that it works on a higher level. It stimulates our higher chakras and thus connects us with the Source. We enter into communication with the spiritual realm and by means of our creativity are able to translate this experience into the physical world. It inspires artistic expression in the new age.

Purification of the higher chakras and stimulation of the third eye are further effects of this essence. It also helps us to get in touch with our spiritual guides, to receive and understand their messages and, finally, to implement them in the physical world. We learn to live and work in communication and harmony with the spiritual world.

Affirmation:
I connect with divine love, and I receive it into myself.

Corresponding gem: Moonstone

LOVE ORCHID
— Oncidium abortivum —

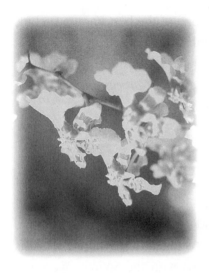

This orchid which grows exclusively on trees is one of the best known *Oncidia*. Its leaves are arranged lengthways. Its delicate yellow flowers shoot out from the axils in large numbers on long panicles. Each flower is shaped like a little angel with a three-cornered hat and a heart chakra which has a special mark.

Love Orchid essence

This could also be called the Healer's Orchid. It represents pure love. It opens the heart chakra and allows the energy of pure love to flow. We become a channel of cosmic love which flows through us like a torrent and can be passed on to others.

It is suitable for those who wish to open their heart chakra and radiate pure love. It is good for healers who wish to improve their work and become a direct channel of cosmic healing love energy.

Affirmation:
I let love flow through me.
I heal myself and I heal others.

Corresponding gem: Rose Tourmaline

PAST LIFE ORCHID
— Paphiopedilum harrysianum —

This orchid has long leaves with rounded tips that grow in the shape of a fan; from their centre springs a single peduncle. For the production of this essence only buds which have just opened are used. They are ovate and hollow.

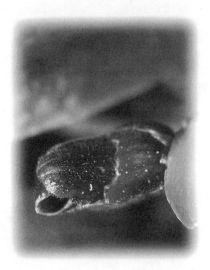

Past Life Orchid essence

This flower bud connects us with other forms of consciousness. We go back into our past and enter the place where all our memories and knowledge are stored. From there we can recall the experience of past lives, finish with self-exploration and move on to getting in touch with true knowledge.

This orchid essence is recommended as a companion for those who wish to work with reincarnation.

Affirmation:
All knowledge is within me and shows me the way.

Corresponding gem: Smoky Quartz

PSYCHE ORCHID
— Paphiopedilum insigne —

The *Paphiopedilum* genus constitutes one of the best known varieties of orchid. Their long leaves rounded off at the tips produce one single flower or several separate flowers with a characteristic slipper-shaped labellum.

Psyche Orchid essence

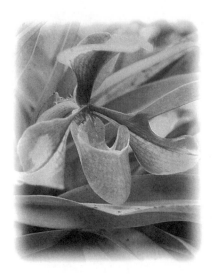

As symbolised by the labellum, this essence allows us to penetrate deeply into ourselves. Who are we really? What is our purpose? Deep inside we find the answer to these questions. This flower essence helps us to find ourselves, to recognise and to accept ourselves. It is the best suited plant to use along with psychotherapy. The main message of this orchid is to allow us to know ourselves and to increase our awareness.

Affirmation:
I am.
I am part of the divine plan.
I am.

Corresponding gem: Amethyst

Sun Orchid
— Epidendrum chioneum —

This terrestrial orchid, which reaches a height of twenty to thirty-five centimetres, is a species that grows on the mountain peaks of Chingaza, an area sacred to the Indians. It grows vertically from the ground.

Sun Orchid essence

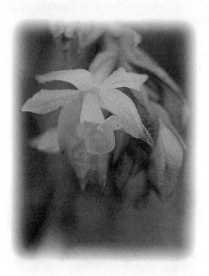

This orchid is anchored in the soil by its roots, just like the chakras of the physical body and, more precisely, the solar plexus, with which it could be identified. We learn to hold ourselves upright just as this plant grows vertically. It opens up the solar plexus which can now connect with the higher chakras and thus allows us to receive the cosmic sun within us. It helps us balance our ego and bring it back into harmony with cosmic law.

Affirmation:
The sun shines within me.
The cosmos and I are one.

Corresponding gem: Rutilated Quartz

VENUS ORCHID
— Anguloa cliftonii —

Long, fan-shaped, linear leaves grow out of its small, stocky bud and the plant grows up to half a metre in height. The yellow or sometimes white flowers appear in ones or twos at the bottom of the leaf stalk. The shape of the flower resembles the female sex organ.

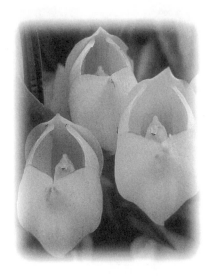

Venus Orchid essence

This orchid is associated with the energies of Venus and the Moon. Its essence allows us to get in touch with subtle feminine energies. It stimulates fertility and the yin in our being and enhances qualities such as listening, understanding, gentleness and love. Mixed in a cream it is gentle and harmonising, and also acts as a tonic for the skin.

Affirmation:
*I accept the feminine part of myself.
I am gentleness and love.*

Corresponding gem: Emerald

VICTORIA REGIA
— Victoria amazonica —

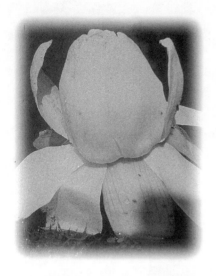

Victoria Regia belongs to the family of *Nymphaeaceae* and is the largest kind of water lily found in the world. Its leaves can grow to a diameter of two metres or more, while its white flowers in comparison are rather small (20-30 cm). It floats on the surface of the lakes and lagoons of Amazonia.

Victoria Regia essence

The flower essence Victoria Regia is full of energy and is similar in this way to the orchid essences. The white lotus-like flower harbours a potent energy, which is reflected on a physical level in its enormous leaves. Its energy, which boosts our own physical energy, is related to the kundalini energy and helps it to rise. It has also been discovered that giving this essence to dying people allows them more easily to adapt their bodily vibrations to the process of dying and helps them to remain conscious and fearless throughout.

Affirmation:
My energies flow freely and lightly.
I have trust and I let go.

Corresponding gem: Ruby

the CENTRE
of the EARTH

THE AMAZON RIVER crosses the South American continent over a distance of five thousand kilometres, parallel to the equator. Its water surface covers seven million square kilometres. With its numerous tributaries and branches it resembles a gigantic tree of life joining the two hemispheres of our planet.

One can compare it with the energetic structure of the human being in whom the central axis dividing the body into two symmetrical parts is represented by the spinal column along which we find the seven chakras linked to the physical body. (The five higher chakras are situated along an invisible extension of this central axis above the head.) The energy surges in through the base chakra, then rises up through the spinal column until, beyond the crown chakra, it reaches the higher chakras which form a large funnel above the head.

Turning our attention now to the structure of our planet Earth, we again find this division into two halves. Starting from the equator which is our planet's axis of symmetry, the various climatic zones with their characteristic vegetation — savannah, steppes and so forth — unfold towards both north and south. Again we see the importance of a central axis on which energetic centres are located.

The Earth rotates fastest at the equator and there receives the strongest cosmic energy. In the tropical rainforests along the length of the equator we find an immense abundance of species and also the largest deposits of gemstones, the highest manifestations of the mineral kingdom. This is the only possible habitat for epiphytic orchids, the highest manifestations of the plant kingdom. Among tropical rainforests Amazonia occupies a special position.

Nowhere else on Earth do we find such a dense occurrence of highly developed life forms as the gemstones, dolphins and orchids of Amazonia. Only today are we beginning to recognise the importance of this region for the health of humans and the entire planet. Because of its characteristics, we can rightly call this area of Amazonia the energetic centre of the Earth. This is why the Amazonian forest, the largest tropical rainforest still in existence, and in effect the heart and lungs of our planet, can be considered the heart chakra of the Earth.

But unfortunately the centre of the Earth is ill. A tropical rainforest is an incredibly complex and highly specialised habitat, and therefore very fragile. As we have seen, its soil mostly consists of a very shallow layer of humus of just eight centimetres. The giant trees have almost no roots anchored in the soil itself and are only supported by stilt-like roots.

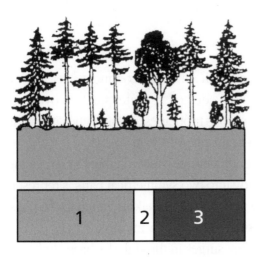

Temperate zones:

Due to the winter cold, organic matter (fallen leaves etc.) only partly decomposes into mineral substance. The soil, only partially decomposed, constitutes a reserve of nutritive material.

1: Soil 2: Decomposing plant matter
3: Living plants

Tropical rainforest:

Organic matter decomposes rapidly. The soil retains only a fraction of it. Approximately 90 per cent of the nutrient reserves are stored in the mass of living plants.

1: Soil
2: Decomposing plants
3: Living plants

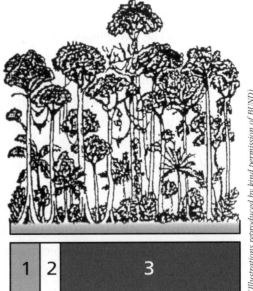

(Illustrations reproduced by kind permission of BUND)

The habitat of Amazonia is becoming increasingly endangered. Through egoism, lust for profit and the human destructive urge, every year an area the size of Germany is felled, burnt and destroyed. The soil is then left unprotected from the heat of the sun, and in no time at all the forces of erosion turn it into a desert.

The Amazon rainforest needs our help!

Nature has less and less space to maintain the energetic balance of our planet, which is our own balance as well. We have subtle bodies that link us with the entire planet and if it gets sick we too feel the effects. We are part of the whole and need to learn to act accordingly.

healing MEDITATION for AMAZONIA

LET US GET IN TOUCH with the centre of the world.by visualising the region of Amazonia.

We now focus our attention on the gemstones and crystals buried underneath the roots of the trees in the soil. We connect with the guardians of the gems. We ask them to send us a lilac-coloured healing light. We imagine the sparkling gemstones and watch them broadcast a light the colour of amethyst. We now see this light spreading further and further into the soil, rising higher and higher, and penetrating to the roots of the trees. We ask the roots of the trees to grow. We see them beginning to grow, becoming stronger and anchoring themselves firmly in the ground.

We watch the lilac-coloured light continue to rise and surround the trees in a protective halo. Now it reaches the orchids that live on the treetops. We visualise these wonderful orchids with their magnificent flowers. We see them on the branches of the trees between the cosmos and the earth. We make contact with the angels of the orchids. We ask them to send forth their light, and we see pink light flow through the orchids from the cosmos onto the earth. We see the pink light of love spreading out and out. Now it joins with the purple light of the gems and flows further and further.

The amethyst and pink light now reaches the Amazon river and spreads over its surface. It makes contact with its most beautiful inhabitants, the dolphins. We feel their joy as they leap out of the water and their cries evoke the connectedness of all life on earth.

Let us give thanks to them for their healing powers.

Now we let the light spread further and further, all the way to the humans who live there. We see how the light reaches the edge of the forest, heals it and rises up like a huge glass wall around the forest. It continues to rise higher and higher and seals Amazonia and its inhabitants beneath a big protective dome of light. All of Amazonia is now bathed in this light.

Now the light spreads even further in all directions. It covers the whole of South America, flows across the oceans, reaches Africa, North America and Asia and the entire surface of the planet. We see the whole Earth bathed in lilac and pink light, a light of purification and of love. Now we send this light to all the spots on earth which require help. To the cities, the people, the oceans and all creatures that need help. The whole Earth is surrounded with light. Now we send this light back to Amazonia, back to the orchids and gemstones, and we thank the guardians of the gems and the angels of the orchids with a powerful vibration of love: OM...

This meditation can be made more powerful by taking Amazonas and Amethyst essences.

APPENDICES

Gem and Orchid Creams

As a complement to taking the essences orally you can also make a corresponding gem or orchid cream. These creams are applied principally to the soles of the feet. In this way the reflex zones that are situated there pass on the necessary energies to all the organs and chakras as well as the subtle plane. You can also apply it directly to the corresponding chakras, lymphatic areas or special points as prescribed.

Basic equipment for making creams

A small pair of scales that can measure grams
A thermometer that goes up to 100° Celsius
A measuring jug for fluids
A small test tube gradated in millilitres
A small heat-proof glass container that can be put into hot water
A glass rod or a plain wooden spoon for stirring
A small pot to heat water
An electric blender with two whisks
A spatula
Containers or jars — preferably of glass and with a capacity of 30 to 50 ml (1–1½ fl.oz.)

Ingredients and tips

Ingredients can be purchased in pharmacies or specialist shops. It is advisable to use products of only the very best quality and to make sure that they are pure and with as little odour as possible, especially in the case of lanolin. Beeswax should be 'natural', in other words yellow. As no preservatives are used, you should only produce small quantities and keep them in the fridge. Jojoba and peanut oil give the cream more stability, but nonetheless you should not keep it any longer than four to six weeks.

Oils

Jojoba is a liquid wax. It is rich in skin-protecting vitamins and has the reputation of being especially gentle to the skin. Peanut oil will keep for a long time, and is rich in vitamins E and F. It is particularly well suited for massage and strengthens one's vitality.

Other ingredients

▶ Beeswax should have a faint smell of honey and is naturally yellow in colour.

▶ Cocoa butter has a pleasant smell and should be bought grated. Keep it refrigerated.

▶ Lanolin and the alcohols of lanolin are the fat of wool with particularly good skin care properties. The anhydride of lanolin should be yellowish and of the best quality, so that it does not smell too strongly. The alcohols of lanolin are hard and it is best to grate them.

▶ Aloe extract 1:1 is an extract of the leaves of the aloe plant. Aloe works in a supporting and purifying way on the subtle level; on the physical level Aloe provides protection against harmful radiation, prevents irritation of the skin and is a valuable aid to treating skin damage. Aloe has a powerful healing effect.

▶ Orange blossom essence is an essential oil and should be of the best quality. It has a calming effect and even extremely sensitive people tolerate it well.

▶ Clear quartz water is an essential ingredient of the creams. Clear quartz with its universal properties is particularly suited for the production of an energised water which has been subtly enriched with silicic acid. Silicic acid purifies the body and has a healing effect. It stabilises the subtle body.

Making clear quartz water

Put the tip of a clear quartz into a stock bottle filled with distilled water. The water can be used after a minimum of 24 hours. The tip of the crystal can remain in the water.

Basic recipe for the cream

4 g beeswax, unbleached
4 g cocoa butter
4 g alcohols of lanolin or an emulsifier
$^1/_2$ teaspoon of anhydride of lanolin, free of pesticides
15 ml jojoba
15 ml peanut oil
45 ml clear quartz water

5 ml aloe extract 1:1
3 drops of orange blossom oil
4 drops of orchid essence
2 drops of gem essence

Melt beeswax, cocoa butter, alcohols of lanolin and lanolin in a pot which is standing in hot water. Add the oils and heat all to 60° Celsius. Heat the clear quartz water together with the aloe extract to 60°C in a separate pot (not aluminium!). Take both off the heat. Mix the water into the hot fat with a blender and add the essences after three minutes without interrupting the process of blending. Keep the blender going until the mass has cooled down and has become a creamy substance. Transfer into containers which have been disinfected and prepared beforehand. This will amount to approximately two small containers of 50 ml (approx. $1^1/_2$ fl. oz.) each. Leave the freshly mixed creams uncapped to cool down.

Various combinations of creams

The gem and orchid essences to be used are indicated by the names of the creams.

▶ **Emerald–Venus Cream**
Strengthens feminine qualities. Understanding, gentleness. Invigorates the skin. To be used as face or neck cream or to be massaged into the reflex zones of the outer ear and the armpits.

▶ **Smoky Quartz–Past Life Cream**
Reflex zone cream to support work with reincarnation. Apply it to the third eye for a meditation aimed at self-knowledge. Suitable for metamorphic technique massage. To be applied locally on the reflex zones of the feet and hands.

▶ **Black Tourmaline–Angel of Protection Cream**
Protection against negative vibrations, especially in cases of depression and worry. For a meditative connection with your guardian angel. Apply on the reflex zones of the feet, and around the navel.

▶ **Olivine–Fun Cream**
For relaxation or when one is depressed or worried. To be applied on the reflex zones of the ears and feet, the armpits and the face.

▶ **Rutilated Quartz–Sun Cream**
To harmonise the chakras. Apply around the navel, on the reflex zones of the feet and on blocked energy centres.

► **Watermelon Tourmaline–Co-ordination Cream**
To be used for cell and skin problems. To enhance the growth of cells. Apply to reflex zones on the face, on the soles of the feet and in the armpits or directly onto affected areas of the skin.

► **Aquamarine–Amazonas Cream**
To get rid of blockages, apply to the relevant areas. Apply to the neck and spine as well, to release tension.

Keywords for the Orchid Essences

Keywords	Orchid
Aggression (unexpressed)	Aggression Orchid
Blockages	Amazonas, Victoria Regia, Aggression Orchid, Sun Orchid
Channelling	Higher Self Orchid, Love Orchid, Deva Orchid, Channelling Orchid
Cell consciousness	Co-ordination Orchid
Children	Venus Orchid
Consciousness	Angel Orchid, Amazonas, Angel of Protection Orchid, Psyche Orchid, Past Life Orchid
Dying	Victoria Regia
Ego	Sun Orchid, Heart Orchid
Energy	Amazonas, Sun Orchid
Femininity	Venus Orchid, Love Orchid
Giving	Horn of Plenty Orchid, Love Orchid
Grounding	Amazonas, Horn of Plenty Orchid
Higher Self	Higher Self Orchid, Channelling Orchid
Joyfulness	Angel Orchid, Fun Orchid, Colour Orchid
Kundalini	Victoria Regia
Life energy	Amazonas, Colour Orchid, Victoria Regia
Listening	Deva Orchid, Channelling Orchid
Love	Heart Orchid, Love Orchid, Chocolate Orchid
Massage	Victoria Regia, Love Orchid, Venus Orchid
Mediumship	Higher Self Orchid, Deva Orchid, Channelling Orchid
Protection	Angel of Protection Orchid
Psychotherapy	Psyche Orchid, Past Life Orchid
Receiving	Horn of Plenty Orchid, Chocolate Orchid, Channelling Orchid
Reincarnation	Past Life Orchid
Safety (security)	Angel Orchid, Angel of Protection Orchid
Self-knowledge	Psyche Orchid, Past Life Orchid
Self-love	Chocolate Orchid
Sexuality	Aggression Orchid, Love Orchid
Transformation	Sun Orchid, Heart Orchid, Co-ordination Orchid, Victoria Regia
Vision	Love Orchid, Higher Self Orchid, Deva Orchid

Orchid	Keywords
Aggression Orchid	Letting go, aggression, sexuality, integration
Amazonas	Connectedness with Earth, flow of energy
Angel Orchid	Communication, heightening of awareness
Angel of Protection Orchid	Need for protection, trust
Channelling Orchid	Communication, integration
Chocolate Orchid	Self-love, opening
Colour Orchid	Joie de vivre, heightening of awareness
Co-ordination Orchid	Cell consciousness, power of self-healing
Deva Orchid	Opening, communication
Horn of Plenty Orchid	Receiving, integrating, giving
Fun Orchid	Serenity, calmness
Heart Orchid	Heightening of consciousness and energy
Higher Self Orchid	Heightening of awareness, exploration of self
Inspiration Orchid	Communication and transformation
Love Orchid	Opening of the heart and healing
Past Life Orchid	Self-exploration, knowledge
Psyche Orchid	Self-discovery, psychotherapy
Sun Orchid	Increase of energy, link with the sun, ego
Venus Orchid	Gentleness, femininity
Victoria Regia	Stimulation, transformation

Indications for the Use of Gem Essences

Gem essence	Physical	spiritual and mental effects
Amazonite	Nerves, muscles	Increased awareness, understanding of nature, abundance of ideas
Amethyst	Migraine, nerves, regulation of sleep	Intuition, meditation spiritual development
Aquamarine	Allergies, vocal cords, language, detoxification of liver, kidneys & lymph	Release of blockages in head and neck, calming of thoughts, light for aura and body
Citrine	Pancreas, diabetes, liver, gall, spleen, digestion, concentration, balancing the two sides of the brain	Tenderness, trust

Clear Quartz	Detoxifying, skin, hair, functioning of bones, stimulation of glands, heart, lungs	Mental order, intuition, connection to Higher Self, light, auric protection
Diamond	Bladder, kidneys, impaired balance, thymus gland, functioning of the whole body	Mental clarity, meditation, gaining awareness, cosmic connectedness, light of the entire spectrum of colours, protection against negativity
Elestial Quartz	Gall, concentration dissolution of anger,	Development, transformation, universal truth, new experience
Emerald	Influenza, stomach, gout, rheumatism, eyes, headaches, diabetes	Self healing powers, love, wisdom, development, meditation, connection to Higher Self
Haematite	Vitality, kidneys, formation of blood, convalescence	Courage for the here and now, self-confidence, being in harmony with oneself
Moonstone	Lymph, detoxification of the body	Creativity, inspiration, understanding
Olivine	Heart, solar plexus, liver, gall, pancreas, spleen	Serenity, joy, mirth
Rose Quartz	Heart, kidneys, liver, lungs, regeneration of kidney tissue, circulatory disorders protection from radiation	Love, opening of heart chakra, trust, love of others, letting go of fears & worries, gentleness,
Ruby	Vitality, heart, reproductive organs	Self love and love for others calming of emotions
Rutilated Quartz	Analgesic, strengthening of thyroid gland, lungs, brain, colds, regeneration of tissue, strengthening of immune system, depression	Stimulation of inspiration, harmony, harmonisation of chakras, light
Smoky Quartz	Abdomen, suprarenal glands, pancreas, muscular degeneration, nerves	Self-responsibility, recognition of one's shadow and purpose, connectedness to Earth
Topaz	Detoxification of the body, strengthening of nerves, glands, digestion	Joie de vivre, happiness
Tourmaline Black	Radiation damage of all kinds, arthritis, disorder of suprarenal glands, asthenia, heart conditions	Dissolution of negativity, protection, terrestrial radiation

Blue	Thyroid gland, lungs, neck problems, expression, language	Connection with higher realms, recognition, knowledge
Rose	Heart trouble, depression	Heartache (sorrow), new beginning, higher knowledge, self-confidence
Watermelon	Disorder of cellular growth (cancer), metabolic disturbances, hormonal disorders	Activation of self-healing powers. This essence should be given in addition to every other essence.

Relationships Between Orchids and Gemstones

Crystal	Orchid
Amazonite	Deva Orchid
Amethyst	Psyche Orchid
Aquamarine	Amazonas
Citrine	Chocolate Orchid
Diamond	Channelling Orchid
Elestial Quartz	Aggression Orchid
Emerald	Venus Orchid
Haematite	Horn of Plenty Orchid
Moonstone	Inspiration Orchid
Olivine	Fun Orchid
Clear Quartz	Higher Self Orchid
Rose Quartz	Heart Orchid
Ruby	Victoria Regia
Rutilated Quartz	Sun Orchid
Topaz	Colour Orchid
Tourmaline (black)	Angel of Protection Orchid
Tourmaline (blue)	Angel Orchid
Tourmaline (rose)	Love Orchid
Tourmaline (watermelon)	Co-ordination Orchid

Orchid	Crystal
Aggression Orchid	Elestial Quartz
Amazonas	Aquamarine
Angel Orchid	Blue Tourmaline
Angel of Protection Orchid	Black Tourmaline
Channelling Orchid	Diamond
Chocolate Orchid	Citrine
Colour Orchid	Topaz
Co-ordination Orchid	Watermelon Tourmaline
Deva Orchid	Amazonite
Fun Orchid	Olivine
Heart Orchid	Rose Quartz
Higher Self Orchid	Clear Quartz
Horn of Plenty Orchid	Haematite
Inspiration Orchid	Moonstone
Love Orchid	Rose Tourmaline
Past Life Orchid	Smoky Quartz
Psyche Orchid	Amethyst
Sun Orchid	Rutilated Quartz
Venus Orchid	Emerald
Victoria Regia	Ruby

The Fund for the Amazon National Park
SENSATION in COLOMBIA!

Discovery of the Valley of the Black Hummingbird

NATURE CONSERVATION organisations in Bogotà were very surprised to learn that a virgin rainforest of an extremely rare type had been discovered 1700 metres up in the Andes in the Virolin valley — the sole survivor of all the rainforests that have been burned and cut down to make way for coffee plantations or grazing pasture.

In the narrow gorges of this misty, almost inaccessible valley grow Humbolt oaks, tropical gnarled oaks and giant ferns. Equally exceptional are its fauna with seventy species of mammal such as the bespectacled bear, the howler monkey and 250 species of bird, some of which are sheer miracles of nature, such as the crested quail and above all the black hummingbird which had been considered extinct.

German organisations devoted to the defence of nature are taking a stand against illegal logging that has started in the Virolin forest and have decided on immediate action:

1. to employ forest rangers to prevent illegal cutting and poaching

2. to establish guard posts to control right of access to the valley

3. to start an awareness-raising campaign aimed at alerting the public to the fact that their future depends upon safeguarding this last virgin rainforest

Since September 1994 we have been carrying on this operation 'Oro Verde', which is a unique opportunity to preserve a biological paradise.

The fund for the Amazon National Park was founded by PHI in order to protect Amazonia. A 15p (25¢) contribution to the Fund will be made by the authors of this book for each copy sold.

Where to find Amazonian Gem and Orchid Essences

The essences are produced by:

▶ Korte PHI Essenzen
   Hauptstrasse 9
   78267 Aach
   Germany
   Tel: +49 (0)7774-7004
   Fax: +49 (0)7774-7009

They are distributed by:

▶ International Flower Essence Repertoire
   The Working Tree
   Milland, Nr Liphook
   Hants GU30 7JS
   UK
   Tel: +44 (0)1428 742 572
   Fax: +44 (0)1428 741 679

▶ Flower Essence Pharmacie
   Gary N Mason
   6600 N Hwy 1
   Little River
   CA 95456
   USA
   Tel: 800-343-8693

ALSO BY FINDHORN PRESS

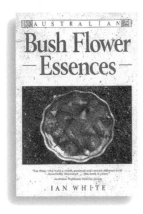

◀ **Australian Bush Flower Essences**
Ian White

ISBN 0 905249 84 4 • Price £11.95 US$19.95

Findhorn Flower Essences ▶
Marion Leigh

ISBN 1 899171 96 7 • Price £9.95 US$16.95

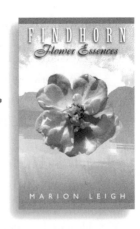

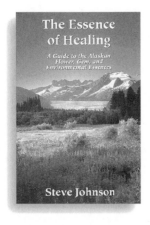

◀ **Alaskan Flower Essences**
(available Spring 1998)
Steve Johnson

ISBN 1 899171 17 7